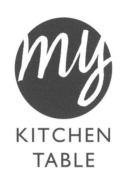

KITCHEN
TABLE

100 Great Low-Fat Recipes

KITCHEN TABLE gives you a wealth of recipes from your favourite chefs. Whether you want a quick weekday supper, sumptuous weekend feast or food for friends and family, let the My Kitchen Table experts bring their favourite dishes to your home.

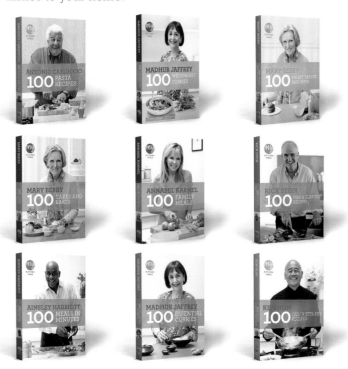

To get exclusive recipes, read our blog, subscribe to our newsletter or find out the latest on our exciting My Kitchen Table recipe App, visit www.mykitchentable.co.uk

Throughout this book, when you see visit our site for practical videos, tips and hints from the My Kitchen Table team.

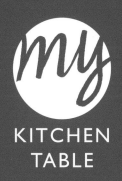

KITCHEN
TABLE

100 Great Low-Fat Recipes

ROSEMARY
CONLEY

www.mykitchentable.co.uk

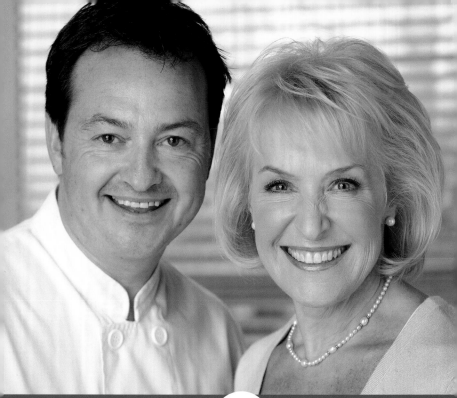

Welcome to my KITCHEN TABLE

Eating low-fat food doesn't mean cutting corners on taste, and here is a collection of **100 exciting recipes that are bursting with flavour but still low in fat**. With delicious dishes like these, eating healthily has never been so easy!

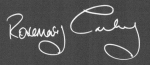

All recipes created by Dean Simpole-Clarke, chef at www.rosemaryconley.tv

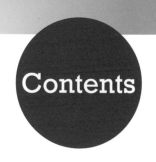

Contents

Soups and starters   6

Poultry   44

Beef, pork and lamb   80

Fish and seafood   116

Vegetables   146

Desserts   178

Index   206

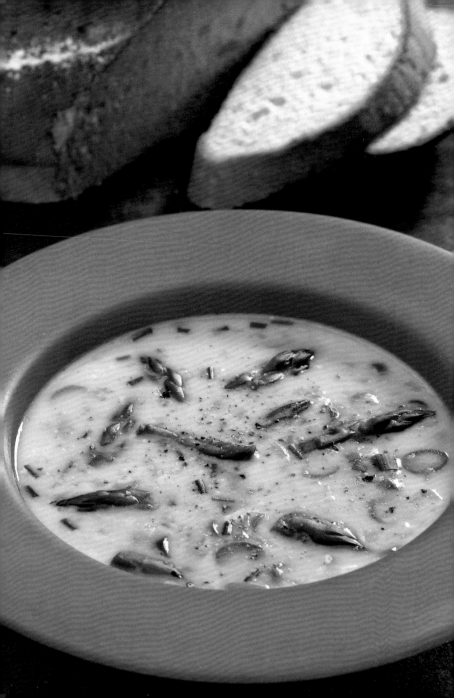

Cream of Asparagus Soup

Asparagus can be bought in many different grades from thick, jumbo stems to the thin, fine spear. Choose thick to medium-thick stems, as the finer stems will disintegrate when cooked over this length of time.

Step one Prepare the asparagus by trimming away the stalk at the point where the stem breaks when snapped in half. Trim off the tips and reserve. Chop the remaining stems into small pieces.

Step two In a non-stick pan, dry-fry the onions over medium heat until soft. Add the garlic and thyme and continue cooking for 1–2 minutes. Add 3 tablespoons of vegetable stock, then sprinkle the flour over and 'cook out' for 1 minute, stirring well with a wooden spoon.

Step three Gradually add the remaining stock, along with the skimmed milk and asparagus stems. Add the bay leaves and gently simmer for 15–20 minutes until the asparagus is just cooked and the soup has slightly thickened.

Step four Five minutes before serving, remove the bay leaves, stir in the asparagus tips and season to taste with salt and black pepper. Serve piping hot and garnished with snipped chives.

Serves 4

225g (8oz) fresh asparagus

2 medium onions, finely chopped

2 garlic cloves, crushed

1 teaspoon chopped fresh thyme

450ml (¾ pint) vegetable stock

1 tablespoon plain flour

450ml (¾ pint) skimmed milk

2 bay leaves

1 tablespoon snipped fresh chives, to garnish

salt and freshly ground black pepper

per serving:

105 kcal/1.3g fat

Sweetcorn and Red Pepper Soup

An easy, colourful soup to brighten up your day. Most of the ingredients can be kept in your store cupboard, making it a quick and easy lunch for all the family.

Serves 4

4 small shallots, finely chopped

1 teaspoon paprika

2 smoked garlic cloves, crushed

2 red peppers, seeded and finely diced

1 x 175g (6oz) tin sweetcorn, drained

pinch of dried chilli flakes

600ml (1 pint) vegetable stock

2 teaspoons cornflour

1 tablespoon finely snipped chives, to garnish

per serving:

50 kcal/1.1g fat

Step one In a large, non-stick pan, dry-fry the shallots over medium heat until soft.

Step two Sprinkle the paprika over, add the garlic and cook for 2–3 minutes, stirring well. Add the peppers, sweetcorn and chilli and stir in the stock. Bring to the boil, then reduce the heat to a gentle simmer.

Step three Slake the cornflour with a little cold water and add to the soup, stirring well to prevent any lumps forming. Cook for 5–6 minutes until the soup thickens slightly. Serve garnished with snipped chives.

If you prefer their flavour, you can use fresh red chillies, very finely chopped, instead of the dried chilli flakes. Use as much or as little as you want, depending on how hot you would like your soup to taste.

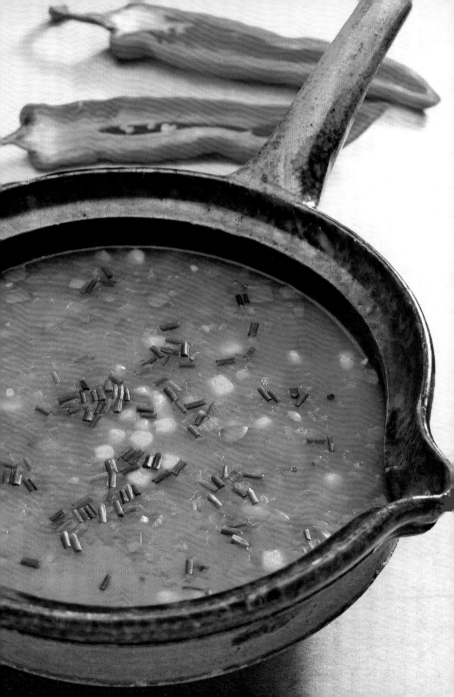

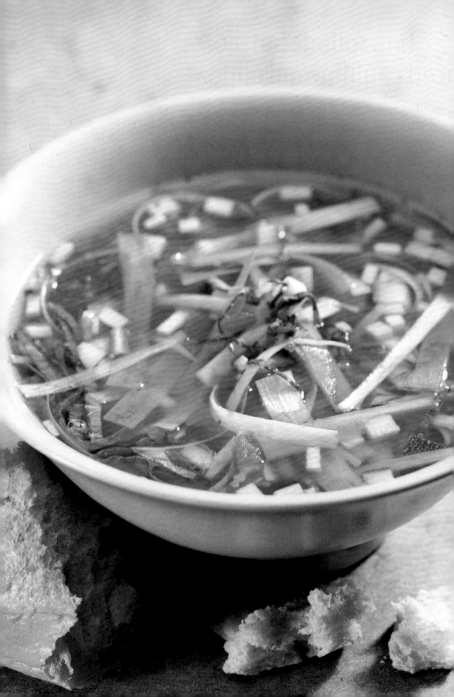

Spring Vegetable Soup

A celebration of fresh, new spring vegetables. Make the soup in advance and reheat as required, adding the spring greens just at the end to prevent them overcooking.

Step one In a non-stick pan, dry-fry the baby leeks, carrots and courgettes for 2–3 minutes over medium heat, until soft but not coloured.

Step two Stir in the stock and chopped tomatoes.

Step three Slake the cornflour with a little water and stir into the soup, bringing the soup up to the boil. Reduce the heat and simmer gently for 10–15 minutes.

Step four Five minutes before serving, add the spring greens and season to taste with salt and black pepper. Serve immediately.

Serves 4

4 baby leeks, finely sliced

2 small carrots, cut into thin strips

2 small courgettes, diced

1.2 litres (2 pints) vegetable stock

1 x 400g (14oz) tin chopped tomatoes

2 teaspoons cornflour

2–3 leaves spring greens, finely chopped

salt and freshly ground black pepper

per serving:

69 kcal/1.4g fat

For a video masterclass on chopping vegetables, go to
www.mykitchentable.co.uk/videos/choppingvegetables

Celeriac and Nutmeg Soup

Celeriac is an unusual root vegetable with a distinctive nutty flavour and is ideal for thick, wholesome winter soups. It can also be boiled with potatoes to add flavour to mashed potatoes.

Serves 4

2 medium
onions, chopped

2 garlic cloves, crushed

450g (1lb) celeriac,
peeled and cut
into chunks

1 tablespoon fresh
chopped thyme

1.2 litres (2 pints)
vegetable stock

fresh nutmeg

3 tablespoons low-fat
fromage frais

flat-leaf parsley,
to garnish

salt and freshly
ground black pepper

per serving:

81 kcal/1.3g fat

Step one Dry-fry the onion and garlic in a non-stick pan over medium heat until soft. Add the celeriac, thyme and stock. Gently simmer for 25–30 minutes until tender.

Step two Pour the soup into a liquidiser or food processor and blend until smooth. Return to the pan, adjusting the consistency with a little more stock if required. Grate over a little fresh nutmeg and season with salt and black pepper. Warm the soup through on medium heat for a few minutes.

Step three Before serving, remove from the heat and stir in the fromage frais. Serve garnished with a sprig of parsley and a little extra grated nutmeg.

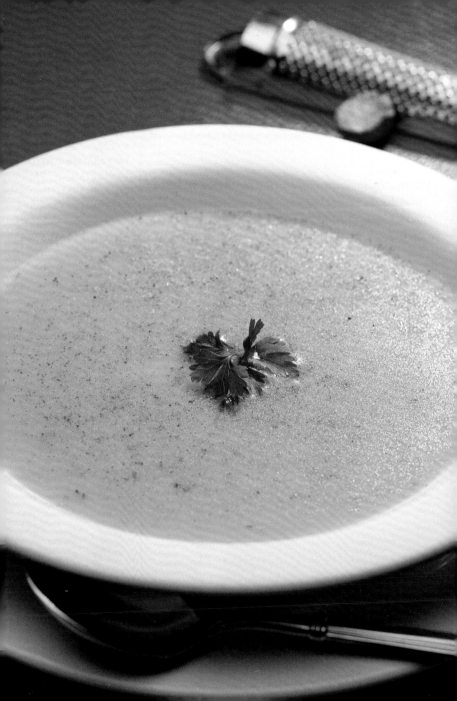

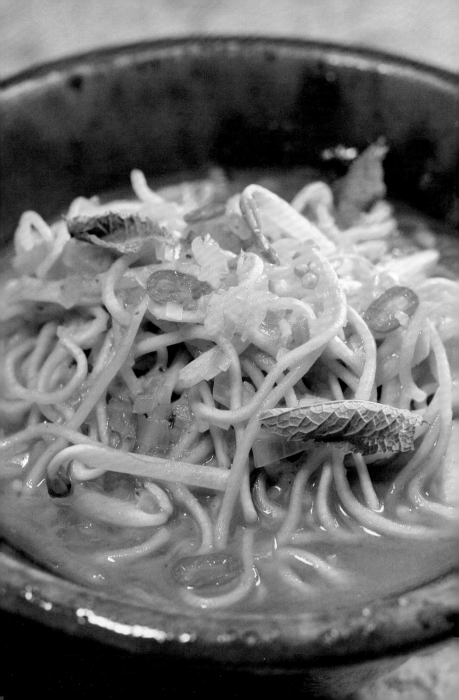

Thai Noodle Soup

Bring the flavours of the Orient to your table with this spicy, wholesome soup. If you find it easier to buy fresh whole spices such as lemon grass or ginger in large quantities, prepare them, and then place in plastic food bags and freeze for later use.

Step one In a large, non-stick pan, dry-fry the shallot over medium heat until soft.

Step two Crush the coriander seeds on a chopping board with the broad side of a chopping knife and add to the pan. Add the garlic and cook for 2–3 minutes, then add the lemon grass, ginger, chilli and turmeric and stir well to combine the spices.

Step three Add the vegetable stock and bring to the boil. Reduce the heat to a gentle simmer and add the noodles. Cook for 5–6 minutes until the noodles become soft, then remove from the heat and stir in the beansprouts and fromage frais.

Step four Just before serving, garnish with mint leaves.

Serves 1

1 small shallot, finely sliced

¼ teaspoon coriander seeds

½ smoked garlic clove, crushed

½ teaspoon lemon grass, finely chopped

small piece fresh ginger, finely chopped

pinch of dried chilli flakes

pinch of ground turmeric

300ml (½ pint) vegetable stock

25g (1oz) egg noodles

25g (1oz) beansprouts

1 tablespoon virtually fat-free fromage frais

mint leaves, to garnish

per serving:
175 kcal/4.1g fat

Watercress and Ginger Soup

This light and refreshing soup is very easy and quick to make. Choose really fresh watercress that is vibrant in colour, perky and with open leaves, as watercress becomes bitter when it starts to wither.

Serves 4

4 baby leeks, finely sliced

2 small carrots, cut into thin strips

225g (8oz) tinned bamboo shoots

1 tablespoon finely chopped fresh ginger

1.2 litres (2 pints) vegetable stock

2 teaspoons cornflour

2 teaspoons light soy sauce

1 bunch watercress

salt and freshly ground black pepper

per serving:

55 kcal/1.5g fat

Step one In a non-stick pan, dry-fry the baby leeks and the carrots for 2–3 minutes over medium heat until soft but not coloured. Stir in the bamboo shoots and fresh ginger, then gradually add the stock.

Step two Slake the cornflour with a little water and stir into the soup. Add the soy sauce and bring the soup to the boil. Reduce the heat and simmer gently for 10–15 minutes.

Step three Remove the tops from the watercress. Just before serving, season the soup to taste with salt and black pepper. Pour into a warmed serving tureen and garnish with the watercress tops.

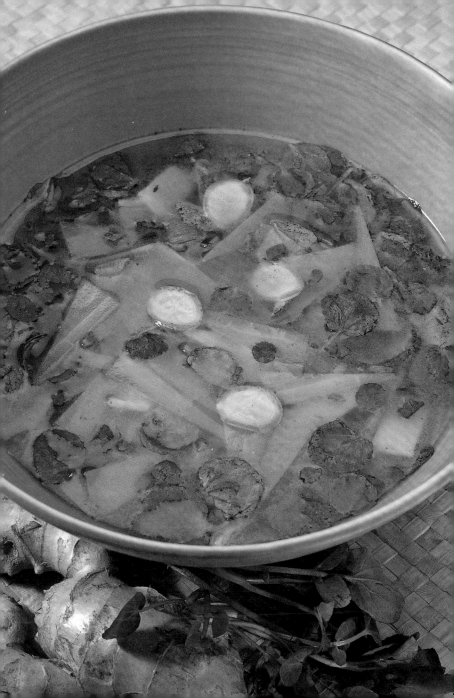

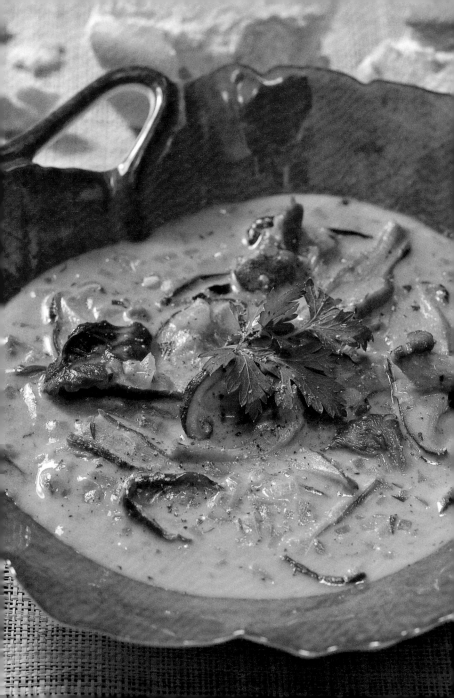

Cream of Wild Mushroom Soup

When buying dried mushrooms, choose good-sized pieces, and avoid broken or shrivelled, dark flakes, as these can be hard and chewy when reconstituted. Fenugreek is a light Indian spice with a slightly nutty taste and is used to flavour curry dishes.

Step one Place the mushrooms, garlic, thyme and stock in a small pan and gently simmer for 10 minutes in order to soften the mushrooms.

Step two In a separate non-stick pan, dry-fry the onions over medium heat until soft. Add the fenugreek and 2 tablespoons of the mushrooms and stock. Sprinkle the flour over and 'cook out' for 1 minute, stirring well with a wooden spoon.

Step three Gradually add the remainder of the mushrooms and stock and the skimmed milk. Add the bay leaves and gently simmer for 20–25 minutes until the mushrooms are soft and the soup has thickened slightly.

Step four Just before serving, remove the bay leaves, stir in the chopped parsley and season to taste with salt and black pepper. Garnish with flat-leaf parsley leaves to serve, if you wish.

Serves 4

40g (1½ oz) good-quality, dried wild mushrooms

2 garlic cloves, crushed

1 teaspoon chopped fresh thyme

450ml (¾ pint) vegetable stock

2 medium onions, finely chopped

¼ teaspoon ground fenugreek

1 tablespoon plain flour

450ml (¾ pint) skimmed milk

2 bay leaves

1 tablespoon chopped fresh flat-leaf parsley, plus extra leaves to garnish (optional)

salt and freshly ground black pepper

per serving:
88 kcal/0.7g fat

Cauliflower and Basil Soup

A winning combination of fresh seasonal flavours. Do not re-boil the soup after it has been liquidised, as this may impair the flavour.

Serves 4

1 large cauliflower

2 medium onions, chopped

1 garlic clove, crushed

600ml (1 pint) vegetable stock

½ teaspoon English mustard powder

2 bay leaves

300ml (½ pint) skimmed milk

20 fresh basil leaves

salt and freshly ground black pepper

per serving:

86 kcal/1.5g fat

Step one Remove and discard the outer leaves from the cauliflower. Coarsely chop the cauliflower, including the stalk, and place in a large pan.

Step two Add the onions, garlic, vegetable stock, mustard powder and bay leaves to the pan. Bring to the boil, then reduce the heat and gently simmer for 15–20 minutes until the vegetables are soft.

Step three Allow to cool slightly, remove the bay leaves, then place the soup in batches in a food processor or liquidiser and liquidise, adding a little of the milk and a few basil leaves to each batch (reserving a few small basil leaves for the garnish), until smooth and lump-free.

Step four Return the soup to the pan and season to taste with salt and black pepper. Adjust the consistency with a little extra milk if required.

Step five Garnish with the reserved basil leaves and serve immediately.

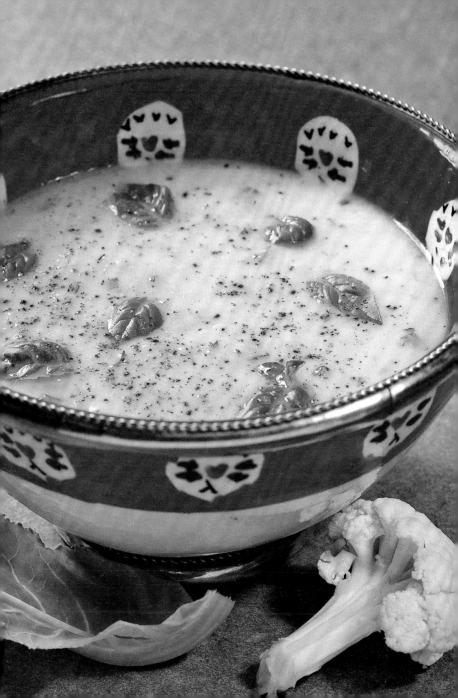

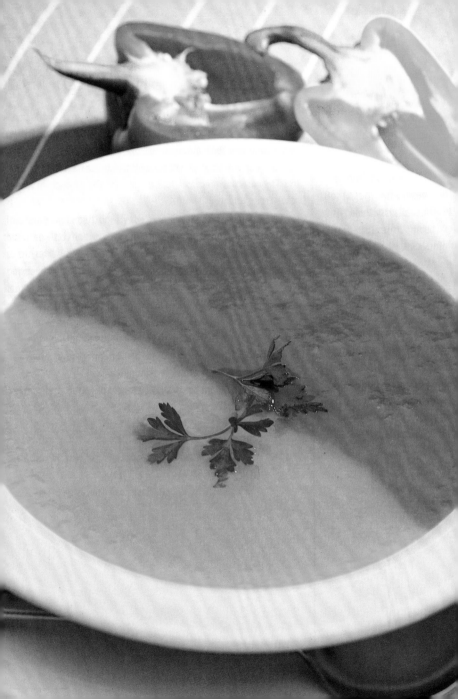

Double Soup of Red and Yellow Peppers

Bring together two vibrant colours in this stunning soup. Use only firm, fresh peppers as these will give a stronger colour to the finished soup. This recipe is excellent for freezing, or the soup can be made in advance and stored in the refrigerator for up to two days.

Step one Using two separate pans, place the red peppers in one and the yellow peppers in the other. Divide all the other ingredients, except the parsley or fromage frais, in half and place half in each pan. Season with salt and black pepper, cover each pan with a lid and simmer for 20–25 minutes or until soft.

Step two Remove the bay leaf from each pan and pour one of the mixtures into a liquidiser or food processor. Blend until smooth, then pour into a clean pan to reheat. Rinse out the liquidiser or food processor and repeat with the second mixture, pouring it into a separate pan when blended.

Step three To serve, pour equal quantities of each soup into two separate jugs. Holding a jug in each hand at either side of a soup bowl, slowly and carefully pour both soups into the bowl at the same time. Garnish with a sprig of parsley or a swirl of fromage frais, if you like.

Serves 4–6

6 red peppers, seeded and chopped

6 yellow peppers, seeded and chopped

2 large onions, chopped

2 garlic cloves, crushed

2 teaspoons chopped fresh thyme

2 celery sticks, chopped

2.5 litres (4 pints) vegetable stock

2 bay leaves

flat-leaf parsley sprig or a little fromage frais, to garnish (optional)

salt and freshly ground black pepper

per serving:
194 kcal/2.3g fat

Crab Bisque

Bring the flavour of the British seaside to your table with this light yet rich crab bisque. For that extra bite, try adding a dash of Tabasco sauce just before serving.

Serves 6

2 medium onions, finely chopped

1 celery stick, finely chopped

600ml (1 pint) fish stock

2 tablespoons flour

150ml (¼ pint) white wine

juice of 1 lemon

225g (8oz) freshly cooked, frozen or tinned crab meat

1 teaspoon anchovy paste

1 tablespoon tomato purée

2–3 tablespoons skimmed milk

½ ladleful brandy

150g (5 oz) low-fat natural yoghurt

chopped fresh parsley, to garnish

salt and freshly ground black pepper

per serving:

113 kcal/1g fat

Step one In a large pan, soften the onions and celery over medium heat in a little fish stock. Add the flour and cook for 1 minute to 'cook out' the flour. Stir in the remaining stock, the white wine and the lemon juice. Simmer for 2–3 minutes until the soup thickens.

Step two Add the crab meat, anchovy paste and tomato purée and cook over low heat for a further 2–3 minutes. If the soup becomes too thick, thin it down with a little skimmed milk.

Step three Heat the brandy in the ladle over a low flame. Tilt the ladle and ignite. Allow the alcohol to burn off the brandy, then pour the brandy into the soup. Season to taste with salt and black pepper, then remove from the heat and stir in the yoghurt. Just before serving, garnish with chopped parsley.

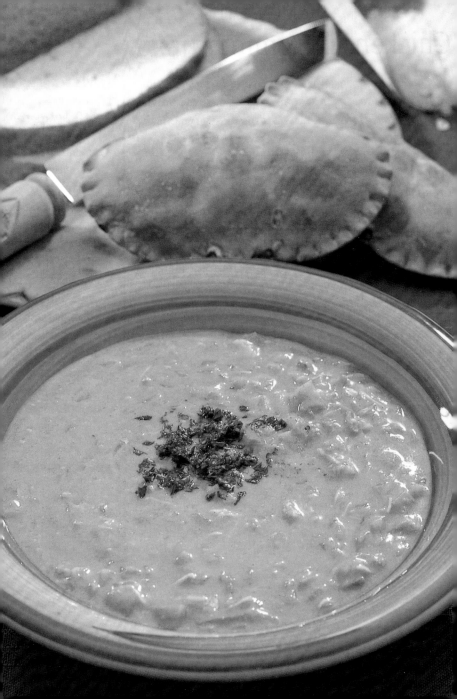

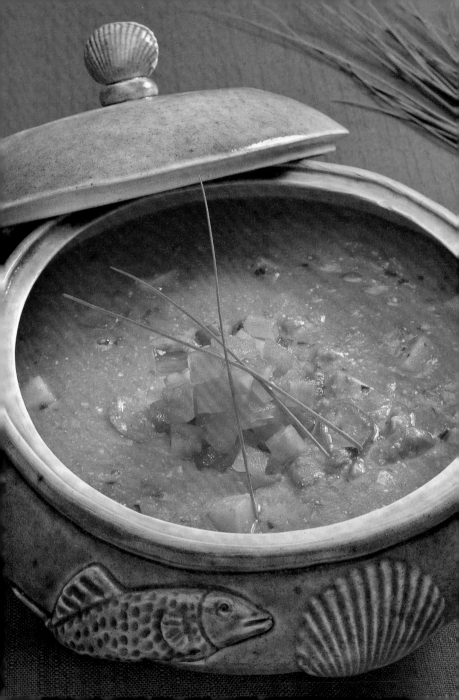

Crab and Tomato Chowder

This is a substantial soup, so it is ideally suited to a lunch.

Step one In a large, non-stick pan, dry-fry the onions over medium heat until soft, add the garlic and 3 tablespoons of the stock. Sprinkle the flour over and beat well with a wooden spoon. Cook for 1 minute in order to 'cook out' the flour, then gradually stir in the remaining stock.

Step two Add the chopped tomatoes, chilli, Passata and potatoes and gently simmer for 10–15 minutes until the potatoes are just cooked.

Step three Stir in the crab meat and herbs and remove the pan from the heat. Add the fromage frais and season to taste with salt and black pepper. Ladle into bowls and garnish with the diced tomato and whole chives to serve.

Serves 4

2 onions, finely chopped

2 garlic cloves, crushed

600ml (1 pint) vegetable stock

2 tablespoons plain flour

1 x 400g (14oz) tin chopped tomatoes

1 small red chilli, seeded and finely chopped

300ml (½ pint) tomato Passata

225g (8oz) small potatoes, peeled and cut into 1cm (½ in) dice

3 dressed crabs, meat removed

1 tablespoon chopped fresh parsley

1 tablespoon snipped fresh chives, plus a few extra whole chives to garnish

2 tablespoons virtually fat-free fromage frais

4 ripe tomatoes, skinned, seeded and diced, to garnish

salt and freshly ground black pepper

per serving:
309 kcal/7.7g fat

27

Smoked Fish and Sweetcorn Chowder

This luxurious soup is ideal for a lunch or you could serve it as a starter, providing you choose a light main course to follow. A chowder is a thick, usually fish, soup thickened with potato and flour. Since smoked fish can sometimes be quite salty, you may need to make your fish stock weak and then add more seasoning once you have added the fish. As a variation, you could add a few cooked prawns.

Serves 4

450g (1lb) smoked haddock or cod

2 onions, chopped

2 tablespoons flour

2 teaspoons English mustard powder

225g (8oz) tinned sweetcorn, drained

225g (8oz) potatoes, peeled and cut into 1cm (½ in) dice

600ml (1 pint) fish stock

300ml (½ pint) skimmed milk

2 tablespoons chopped fresh parsley

fish-stock cube, optional

2 tablespoons virtually fat-free fromage frais

salt and freshly ground black pepper

per serving:
252 kcal/2.04g fat

Step one Place the fish in a pan. Add 600ml (1 pint) water and simmer for 10 minutes until tender. Strain, reserving the liquid. Flake the fish coarsely, discarding any skin and bones.

Step two Dry-fry the onions over medium heat in a large, non-stick pan until soft. Add 3 tablespoons of the reserved liquid, sprinkle the flour over and beat well with a wooden spoon. Cook for 1 minute in order to 'cook out' the flour. Gradually add the remainder of the reserved liquid, stirring continuously.

Step three Add the mustard powder, sweetcorn and potatoes, stock and milk. Bring to the boil, reduce the heat and simmer for 10 minutes until the vegetables are tender.

Step four Stir in the flaked fish and the parsley. Taste, and adjust the seasoning with a fish-stock cube, if necessary, and salt and black pepper. Just before serving, stir in the fromage frais. Serve piping hot.

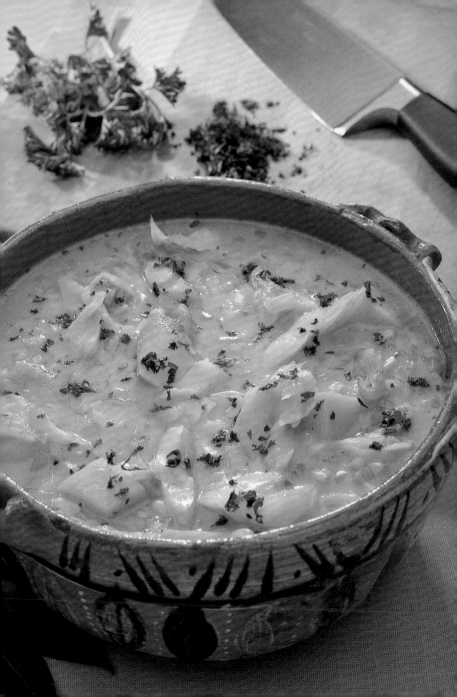

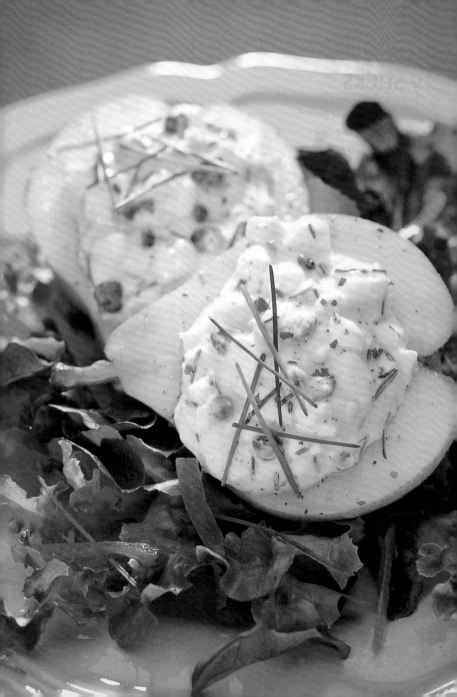

Lemon- and Caper-stuffed Pears

Choose good round pears such as Williams or Doyenné du Comice. They need to be firm but ripe for this dish to be at its best.

Step one Peel the pears, cut each one in half and scoop out the cores with a teaspoon or melon-baller. Using the point of a small knife, ease out the part leading to the stalk. Brush the lemon juice all over the pears.

Step two Mix together the cottage cheese, capers and 1 tablespoon of the snipped chives and season with salt and black pepper. Place a good spoonful in the centre of each pear. Place a leaf or two of Lollo Rossa on each of four individual plates and place two pear halves in the centre of each. Cover and chill until required.

Step three Just before serving, sprinkle the crushed red peppercorns and the remaining snipped chives over the top of the cottage-cheese mixture.

Serves 4

4 large ripe pears

2–3 tablespoons lemon juice

175g (6oz) low-fat cottage cheese

1 tablespoon capers

1–2 tablespoons snipped chives

1 small Lollo Rossa lettuce

1 teaspoon crushed red peppercorns

salt and freshly ground black pepper

per serving:

132 kcal/0.8g fat

Marinated Roast Vegetables

These marinated roast vegetables are a perfect light starter. Serve them piping hot from the oven or chilled with salad leaves. Either way, the strong, contrasting flavours make this such a tasty dish.

Serves 4

2 medium courgettes

1 aubergine

1 red and 1 yellow pepper, seeded

2 baby leeks

1 small bulb fennel

1 red onion

4 tablespoons lemon juice

2 tablespoons light soy sauce

2 teaspoons finely chopped lemon grass

2 tablespoons chopped fresh marjoram

1 tablespoon sesame seeds

chopped fresh parsley, to garnish

salt and freshly ground black pepper

per serving:

79 kcal/2.6g fat

Step one Prepare the vegetables by slicing into wedges about 1cm (½in) thick. Place in a roasting tin and season well with salt and black pepper.

Step two Combine the lemon juice, soy sauce, lemon grass and marjoram in a small bowl. Pour the mixture over the vegetables and allow the vegetables to marinate for at least 30 minutes, turning occasionally.

Step three Preheat the oven to 200°C/400°F/gas 6. Give the vegetables a final mix, sprinkle with the sesame seeds and place in the oven. Roast for 35–40 minutes until soft and tender with slight charring around the edges. Serve garnished with a sprinkling of chopped parsley.

For more recipes from My Kitchen Table, sign up for our newsletter at www.mykitchentable.co.uk/newsletter

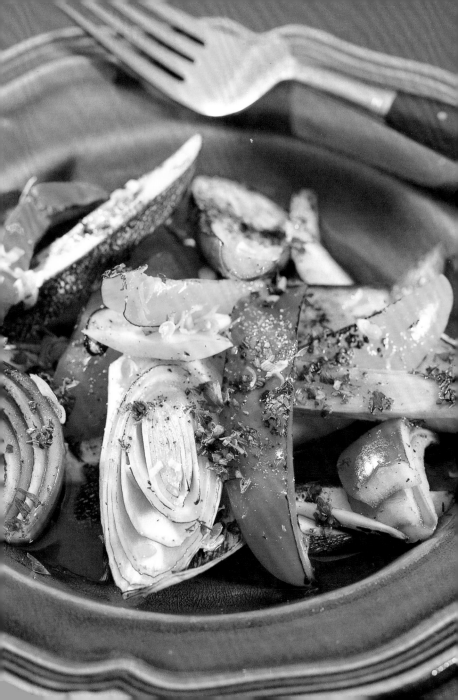

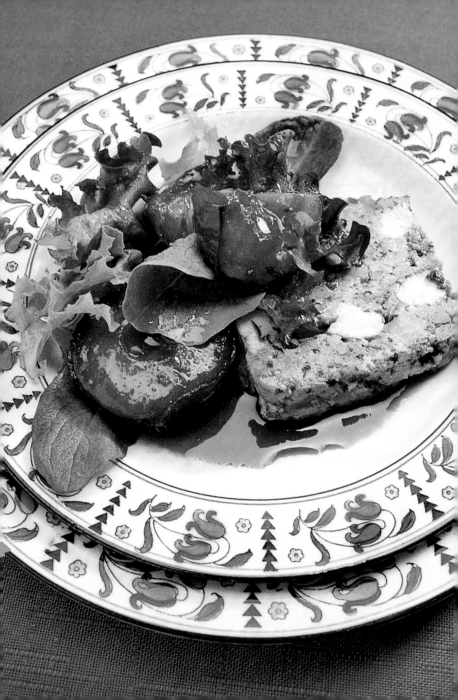

Pork and Chicken Pâté with Spiced Plums

This coarse, dense and meaty pâté uses only lean ingredients to cut down on fat. The spicy, syrupy plums form the perfect accompaniment.

Serves 10

Step one Preheat the oven to 180°C/350°F/gas 4. Roughly chop the chicken livers and place in a large bowl with the minced pork. Add the garlic, peppercorns, herbs, brandy and stock. Season well with salt and black pepper and mix to combine.

Step two Cut the chicken breasts into thin strips. Place a thin layer of the chicken-liver and pork mixture in a 900g (2lb) non-stick loaf tin, just enough to cover the base. Add a third of the sliced chicken. Continue with additional layers, ending with the chicken-liver and pork mixture. Cover with foil.

Step three Set the loaf tin in a roasting tin. Pour sufficient water in the roasting tin to come halfway up the sides of the loaf tin and place in the oven for 1½ hours.

Step four When cooked, remove the pâté from the oven. Allow to cool, and then chill overnight.

Step five To make the spiced plums, dissolve the sugar in the cider vinegar over low heat, then add the spices, lemon juice, zest and salt. Cut the plums in half, remove the stones, then add to the pan, cover, and gently simmer for 15 minutes. Remove from the heat and allow to cool, still covered. Pour into a container and chill until ready for use.

Step six To serve, slice the pâté thinly and garnish with the spiced plums and the salad leaves.

For the best results, always use fresh, dark Victoria plums to make the spiced plums. These spiced plums taste delicious served with any cold meats or spicy foods and will keep in the refrigerator for up to two weeks.

225g (8oz) chicken livers

450g (1lb) lean minced pork

2 garlic cloves, crushed

8 green peppercorns

1 tablespoon chopped fresh flat-leaf parsley

2 tablespoons chopped fresh mixed herbs (tarragon, chervil, chives)

2 tablespoons brandy

150ml (¼ pint) cool vegetable stock

2 skinless chicken breasts

salad leaves, to garnish

salt and freshly ground black pepper

for the spiced plums

115g (4oz) soft dark brown sugar

150ml (¼ pint) cider vinegar

2 teaspoons coriander seeds

⅓ teaspoon allspice

juice and zest of 1 lemon

pinch of sea salt

450g (1lb) plums

per serving:
187 kcal/5.5g fat

Sweet Potato and Red Pepper Terrine

A stunning starter, this vegetarian pâté is also suitable for picnics and lunchboxes. Roasting the peppers is time-consuming, but it does add a much stronger flavour to the dish. Once cooled, the terrine will keep in the refrigerator for four to five days.

Serves 6

3 red peppers, cut in half and seeded

900g (2lb) sweet potatoes, peeled

grated fresh nutmeg, to taste

2 garlic cloves, crushed

1 tablespoon chopped fresh mixed herbs

2 tablespoons tomato purée

2 eggs

mixed salad leaves, to serve

salt and freshly ground black pepper

per serving:

186 kcal/2.7g fat

Step one Preheat the oven to 180°C/350°F/gas 4.

Step two Place the peppers, skin-side up, on a baking tray and grill under a high heat until the skins start to blacken and blister. Place the peppers inside a plastic food bag and seal to make airtight. Once cool, remove the peppers, peel away the skins and cut into small dice.

Step three Cut the sweet potatoes into large chunks and cook in a pan of boiling salted water until soft. Drain well and mash until smooth, seasoning with grated nutmeg and black pepper.

Step four Mix the garlic, herbs and tomato purée with the potatoes, then beat in the eggs one at a time. Fold in the diced red pepper and spoon into a 600ml (1 pint) terrine mould or loaf tin.

Step five Place the terrine in a roasting tin and pour in enough boiling water to come halfway up the sides of the terrine mould or loaf tin. Bake in the oven for 45 minutes. Allow to cool and chill until ready to serve.

Step six Turn out onto a large plate. Slice the terrine and place one or two slices per person on a bed of mixed salad leaves.

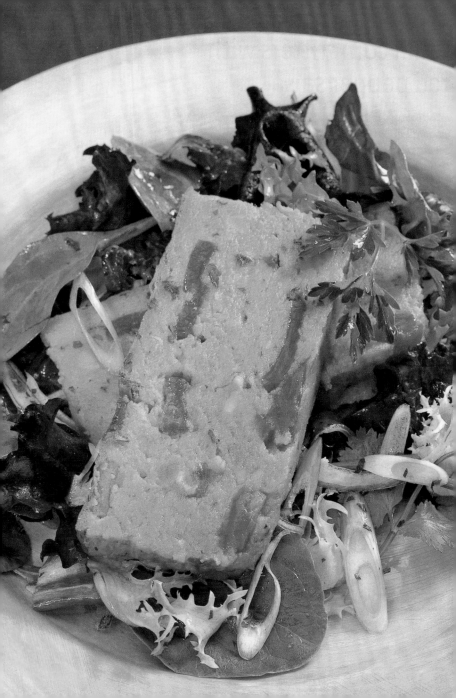

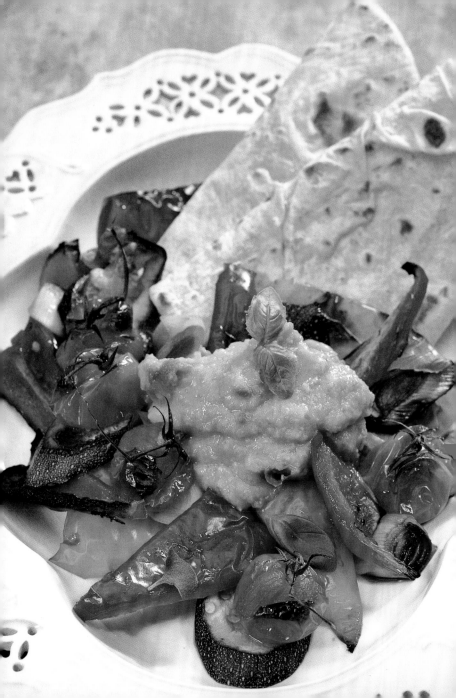

Sun-dried Tomato Hummus with Roasted Summer Vegetables

Hummus is a garlic-spiked chickpea paste, usually made with a large quantity of highly fattening oil. In this recipe, the tomatoes add colour and a sweet flavour, making it much lighter to eat. Squeezing a little fresh lemon juice over the hummus adds that extra touch.

Step one Preheat the oven to 200°C/400°F/gas 6.

Step two Place all the vegetables, along with the chopped rosemary and basil leaves, in a roasting tin and drizzle with the soy sauce. Roast in the top of the oven for 20–25 minutes, turning occasionally. Allow to cool.

Step three In a pan, heat the milk with the sun-dried tomatoes and garlic over medium heat until hot but not boiling. Reduce the heat and simmer for 8–10 minutes until the tomatoes have softened. Allow to cool.

Step four Drain and rinse the chickpeas and place in a food processor. Pour in the milk mixture and process until smooth. Season with lots of salt and black pepper, then add the lemon juice and blend again to combine. Adjust the consistency with a little extra milk if required.

Step five To serve, arrange the cooled vegetables on plates, placing a spoonful of hummus in the centre of each.

Stored in the refrigerator, this light version of traditional hummus will keep for five days.

Serves 4

for the roasted vegetables

2 baby courgettes, sliced

2 red and 2 yellow peppers, seeded and cut into chunks

3 baby leeks, sliced

8 small vine tomatoes

1 teaspoon chopped fresh rosemary

a handful of fresh basil

2 tablespoons light soy sauce

for the hummus

300ml (½ pint) skimmed milk

3–4 pieces sun-dried tomato (dried rather than type stored in oil)

2 garlic cloves, crushed

1 x 410g (14oz) tin chickpeas with no added salt or sugar

juice of 1 lemon

salt and freshly ground black pepper

per serving:
230 kcal/6.2g fat

Blinis with Smoked Salmon and Horseradish Cream

Blinis are light, batter pancakes often used as a canapé or starter to serve as a base for salmon or caviar. Our low-fat version can be made in different sizes to suit. For a neat, uniform look use a round pastry cutter to trim them to equal size.

Serves 6

for the blinis

300ml (½ pint) skimmed milk

15g (½ oz) fresh or dried yeast

175g (6oz) plain flour

75g (3oz) buckwheat flour

1 egg yolk

75g (3oz) virtually fat-free fromage frais

4 egg whites

pinch of salt

a little vegetable oil for the pan

for the topping

115g (4oz) smoked salmon

4 tablespoons virtually fat-free fromage frais

1 teaspoon horseradish sauce

fresh dill sprigs, to garnish

salt and freshly ground black pepper

per serving:
226 kcal/2.7g fat

Step one Warm the milk to a temperature that's no more than hand-hot. Add the yeast and whisk well.

Step two Combine the two flours in a mixing bowl, add the egg yolk and fromage frais, then, using a whisk, gradually pour in the milk, beating the mixture to a smooth, lump-free batter. Allow to stand and prove for 30 minutes.

Step three Whisk the egg whites with a pinch of salt to stiff peaks, then carefully fold into the batter with a metal spoon.

Step four Preheat a non-stick frying pan over medium heat, then lightly oil the pan, removing any excess with kitchen paper. Spoon tablespoons of the batter separately into the pan and cook for 1 minute, then flip over and cook the other side for a further 2 minutes. Allow to cool on a wire rack.

Step five Place the blinis on a serving plate and drape the smoked salmon on top. Mix together the fromage frais and horseradish sauce, seasoning well with salt and black pepper, and spoon on top. Garnish with fresh dill.

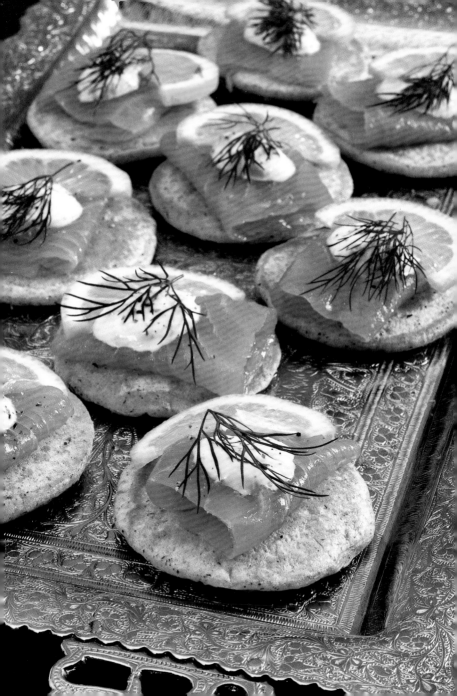

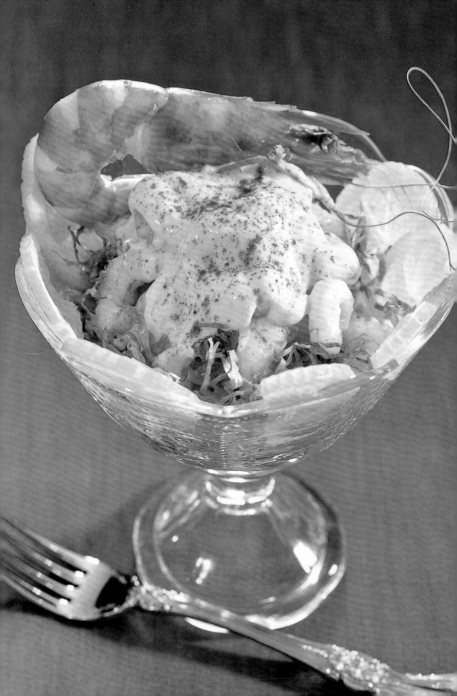

Prawn Cocktail

Recreate this classic starter using low-fat ingredients. The sauce can also be used on many other seafood dishes or can be served with cold crab or lobster.

Step one Wash the prawns and drain well. Wash the lettuce leaves, drain well and finely shred. Place the shredded lettuce in the bottom of four wine glasses or small dishes and arrange the prawns on top.

Step two Combine the tomato ketchup, yoghurt and salad dressing in a small bowl, and season to taste with salt and black pepper and a dash of Tabasco sauce. Spoon the dressing over the prawns and sprinkle with paprika. Garnish with lemon slices.

Serves 4

350g (12oz) peeled and cooked prawns

1 crisp green lettuce

4 tablespoons tomato ketchup

4 tablespoons low-fat natural yoghurt

2 tablespoons reduced-oil, low-calorie salad dressing

dash of Tabasco sauce

paprika

4 lemon slices, to garnish

salt and freshly ground black pepper

per serving:
122 kcal/1.2g fat

Chicken Caesar Salad

Traditionally, Caesar salad is served with an exceptionally high-fat dressing and deep-fried croutons. In this low-fat version, the chicken brings flavour and texture and the low-fat dressing tastes delicious.

Serves 4

4 boneless, skinless chicken breasts

1 Romaine lettuce or iceberg lettuce, shredded

4 spring onions, sliced

½ cucumber, cut into batons

flat-leaf parsley sprigs, to garnish

for the dressing

4 tablespoons low-fat salad dressing

1 tablespoon virtually fat-free fromage frais

1 garlic clove, crushed

fresh lemon juice, to taste

salt and freshly ground black pepper

per serving:

138 kcal/5.8g fat

Step one Preheat a non-stick frying pan over medium-high heat. Cut the chicken into strips and season well with salt and black pepper. Place in the pan and cook briskly, turning regularly, for 8–10 minutes.

Step two Place the shredded lettuce in a large bowl. Add the spring onions and cucumber, toss well and arrange on a serving dish.

Step three Combine the dressing ingredients in a small bowl. Place the cooked chicken on the salad, drizzle the dressing over and garnish with flat-leaf parsley sprigs.

Vegetarians may use dry-fried courgettes instead of chicken.

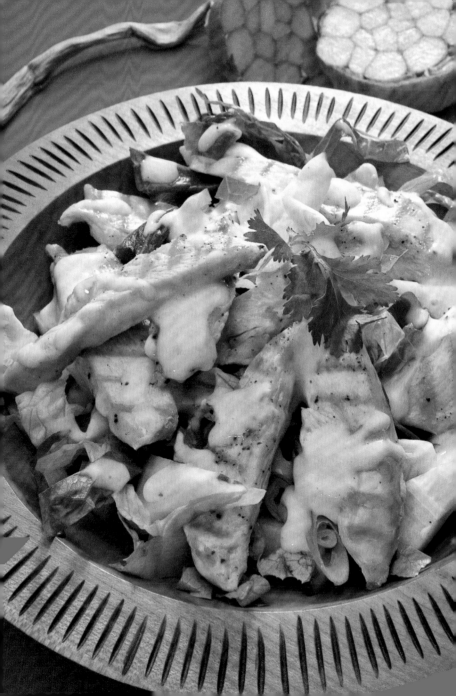

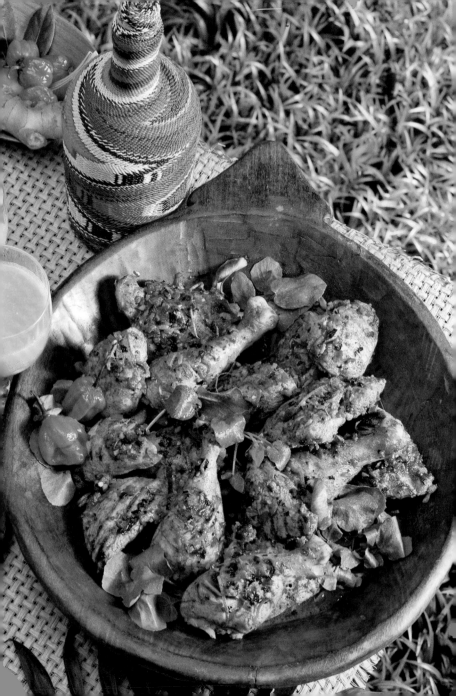

Jamaican Jerk Chicken

There are many variations of this spicy, flavoursome chicken dish. This one uses Habanero or Scotch Bonnet chillies, some of the hottest chillies available. If your palate doesn't stretch to this heat scale, then substitute with a milder bullet variety or play safe with a little chilli sauce.

Step one Prepare the chicken by removing all traces of fat and any white strands of sinew. Slash the flesh of each piece with a sharp knife several times and place in a non-metallic bowl. Season each piece well with salt and black pepper.

Step two Prepare the jerk seasoning by crushing the allspice berries either in a pestle and mortar or by using the broad edge of a large chopping knife, pressing the berries against a solid chopping board. Place in a small glass bowl and add the red onion and garlic. Add the remaining jerk seasoning ingredients and mix well. Spread the mixture over the chicken, turning each piece to coat. Allow to marinate for 2–3 hours.

Step three Cook the chicken either under a preheated hot grill or on a barbecue for approximately 20–25 minutes. It is very important to check that the chicken is fully cooked through to the centre before serving. The juices should run clear when a knife is inserted into the thickest part of the chicken.

Step four Just before serving, sprinkle with chopped coriander. Serve hot or cold with rice and a selection of salads.

Serves 4

8 pieces skinless chicken (drumstick, breast or thighs)

2 tablespoons chopped fresh coriander, to garnish

salt and freshly ground black pepper

for the jerk seasoning

6–8 allspice berries

1 small red onion, finely chopped

2 garlic cloves, crushed

1 teaspoon finely chopped fresh ginger

½ teaspoon ground mace

Habanero or Scotch Bonnet chilli, finely chopped

2 tablespoons light soy sauce

zest and juice of 3 limes

per serving:
396 kcal/5.8g fat

For a video masterclass on using a pestle and mortar, go to
www.mykitchentable.co.uk/videos/pestlemortar

Thai Chicken Breasts

Oil and coconut milk are common ingredients in Thai cookery. This fruity recipe gives the flavour of Thai cooking without the fat.

Serves 4

4 boneless chicken breasts, skinned

1 red pepper, seeded and finely sliced

6 spring onions, finely chopped

6 plum tomatoes, skinned, seeded and diced

1 green chilli, seeded and finely chopped

zest and juice of 2 limes

2 garlic cloves, crushed

1 teaspoon ground cumin

1 teaspoon ground coriander

1 tablespoon cornflour

300ml (½ pint) pineapple juice

chopped fresh coriander, to garnish

salt and freshly ground black pepper

per serving:
204 kcal/7.4g fat

Step one Preheat the oven to 190°C/375°F/gas 5.

Step two Place the chicken in an ovenproof dish and season well on both sides with salt and black pepper.

Step three Place the red pepper, spring onions and tomatoes in a bowl. Add the chilli, lime juice and zest, garlic, cumin and coriander and combine well. Dissolve the cornflour in the pineapple juice and pour over the vegetables. Mix well and season with plenty of salt and pepper. Pour over the chicken and bake for 30–35 minutes.

Step four Garnish with coriander and serve with jasmine rice.

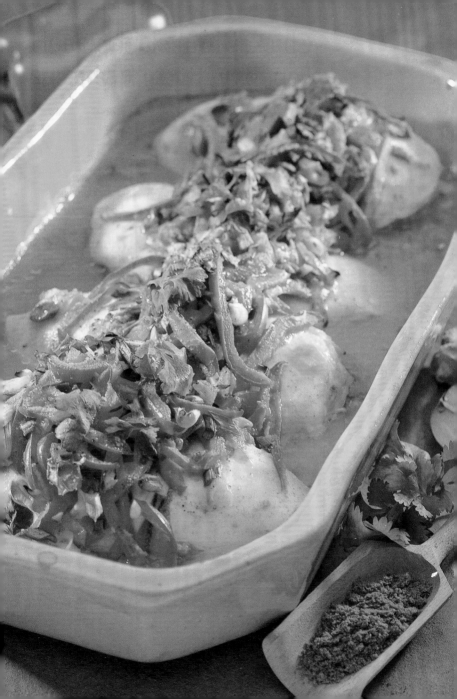

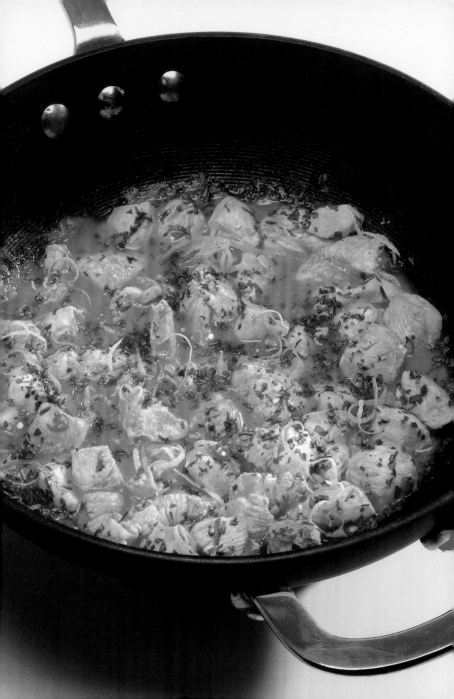

Spicy Lemon Chicken

A great family chicken dish. Lemon grass is available fresh or dried, but using fresh will enhance the flavour of the finished dish.

Step one Using a sharp knife, cut the chicken breasts into dice and place in a shallow dish. Season with salt and black pepper. Combine the remaining ingredients, except the fresh coriander, and pour over the chicken. Leave to marinate for at least 1 hour, mixing occasionally.

Step two Strain the marinade from the chicken and reserve. Heat a non-stick wok or frying pan over high heat and dry-fry the chicken quickly for 5–6 minutes, turning it to seal all of the sides.

Step three Add the reserved marinade, reduce the heat and continue to cook for a further 10 minutes, to allow the sauce to simmer gently and thicken. Sprinkle over the chopped coriander and serve.

Serves 4

450g (1lb) boneless, skinless chicken breast

zest and juice of 1 lemon

2 tablespoons light soy sauce

1 teaspoon ground coriander

150ml (¼ pint) tomato Passata

1 small red chilli, finely sliced

1 teaspoon finely chopped lemon grass

2 garlic cloves, crushed

1 tablespoon chopped fresh coriander, to garnish

salt and freshly ground black pepper

per serving:

146 kcal/2.5g fat

Stuffed Chicken Breasts

These mini chicken roulades make a good main course for a dinner party.

Serves 4

4 x 100g (4oz) boneless, skinless chicken breasts

¼ small red pepper

¼ small green pepper

¼ large carrot

1 medium onion

6 medium white mushrooms

1–2 tablespoons low-fat fromage frais

1 tablespoon chopped fresh coriander or tarragon

2–3 teaspoons lemon juice

300ml (½ pint) chicken stock

for the sauce

300ml (½ pint) skimmed milk

15g (½ oz) cornflour

salt and freshly ground black pepper

per serving:

224 kcal/6.2g fat

Step one Preheat the oven to 180°C/350°F/gas 4. Remove the fillet from the back of each chicken breast and, using a sharp knife, scrape out the thick sinew and discard. Reserve the fillets. Place the chicken breasts on a chopping board and cut through each breast from the thick side until you can open it out like an escalope. Place a fillet in the centre of each breast, cover with a piece of clingfilm, then hammer the chicken out gently using a rolling pin.

Step two Chop the vegetables finely, without mixing them up, and place half in a bowl. Add sufficient fromage frais to bind them plus half the coriander or tarragon. Season and then place a tablespoon of vegetables on each breast, roll up, and secure each one with a small skewer or cocktail stick.

Step three Place each chicken roll on a piece of foil. Season lightly and sprinkle with lemon juice. Seal each tightly in the foil and place in a roasting tin. Bake for 35–45 minutes until tender.

Step four Cook the remainder of the vegetables, except the mushrooms, over medium heat in the stock. When most of the liquid has gone, add the mushrooms and cook for 2–3 minutes.

Step five When the chicken is done, make a white sauce: pour a little of the milk onto the cornflour and mix well. Heat the remainder of the milk in a pan until hot but not boiling. Pour a little hot milk onto the cornflour mixture, stirring continuously. Slowly stir in the remainder of the milk. Mix well and return to the pan with any residual stock from the vegetables. Stirring continuously, bring to the boil, and cook for 2–3 minutes.

Step six Add the vegetables and the remaining herbs. Season, then remove the chicken from the foil and take out the skewers or cocktail sticks. Place the breasts on a hot serving dish, pour a little of the sauce over and serve the rest separately.

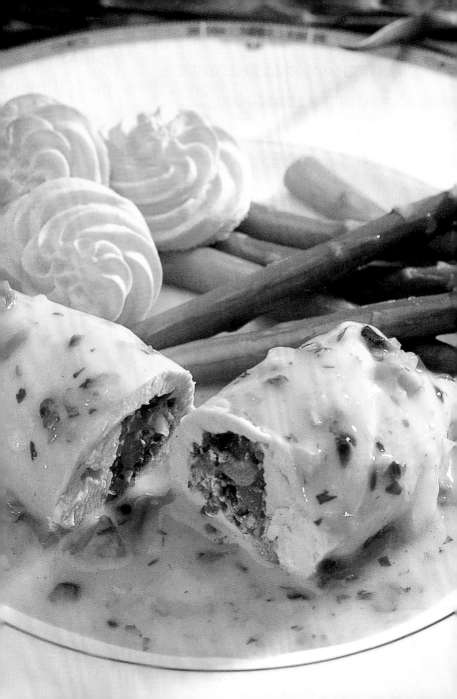

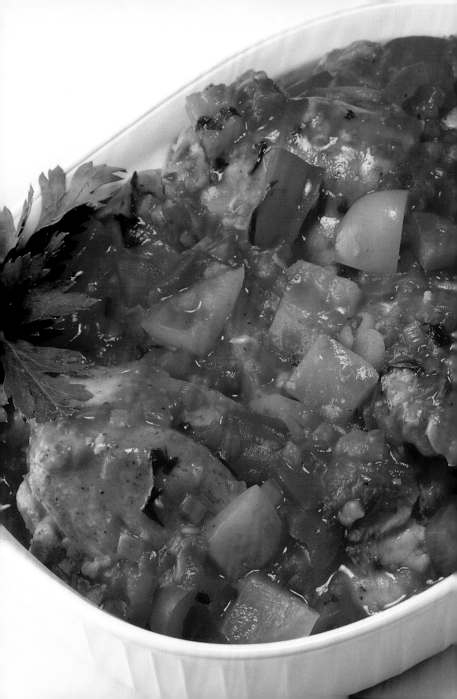

Chicken Casserole with Peppers

This recipe works equally well with lean pork steaks or even turkey-breast fillets. The white wine may be substituted with cider or apple juice.

Step one Preheat a non-stick pan over medium heat. Add the onion and dry-fry until soft.

Step two Season the chicken on both sides and add to the pan, lightly browning on each side. Remove the chicken from the pan and keep warm.

Step three Add the garlic and 2 tablespoons of stock to the onion. Stir in the flour and 'cook out' for 1 minute. Add the remaining stock, the wine and tomatoes, followed by the tarragon and peppers, and bring to the boil.

Step four Return the chicken to the pan and cover with a lid. Gently simmer for 30–35 minutes. Sprinkle with chopped parsley and garnish with a few sprigs to finish and serve with seasonal vegetables.

Serves 4

1 medium onion, finely chopped

1 chicken, jointed with skin removed

2 garlic cloves, crushed

150ml (¼ pint) chicken stock

2 tablespoons plain flour

3 tablespoons dry white wine

1 x 400g (14oz) tin chopped tomatoes

1 tablespoon chopped fresh tarragon

1 red pepper, diced

1 yellow pepper, diced

1 tablespoon chopped fresh parsley, plus a few sprigs, to garnish

salt and freshly ground black pepper

per serving:
304 kcal/4.7g fat

Thai Chicken Curry

Marinating the chicken overnight maximises the flavour of this very spicy curry. Once cooked, the finished curry can be stored chilled or frozen and reheated as required.

Serves 4

for the paste

3 garlic cloves

1 tablespoon ground coriander

½ teaspoon ground turmeric

½ teaspoon fenugreek seeds or ground fenugreek

2–3 small whole fresh chillies

seeds removed from 4 crushed cardamom pods

for the chicken curry

4 large boneless, skinless chicken breasts, cut into pieces

1 large red onion, finely chopped

2 tablespoons tomato purée

600ml (1 pint) chicken or vegetable stock

1 tablespoon tamarind paste or hot fruit chutney

4 kaffir lime leaves

2 tablespoons chopped fresh coriander

Step one First, make the paste by grinding all the ingredients in either a food processor or liquidiser.

Step two Scrape the paste into a bowl, then rinse out the food processor bowl with a little stock. Add the chicken pieces to the paste and mix well. Allow to marinate for a minimum of 1 hour or ideally overnight.

Step three In a non-stick pan over medium heat, dry-fry the onion until soft, then add the chicken and cook for 5–6 minutes, stirring continuously. Add the remaining ingredients except the fresh coriander, lower the heat and simmer gently for 15–20 minutes, until the sauce thickens and the chicken is fully cooked through.

Step four Just before serving, stir in the fresh coriander.

per serving:

240 kcal/3.3g fat

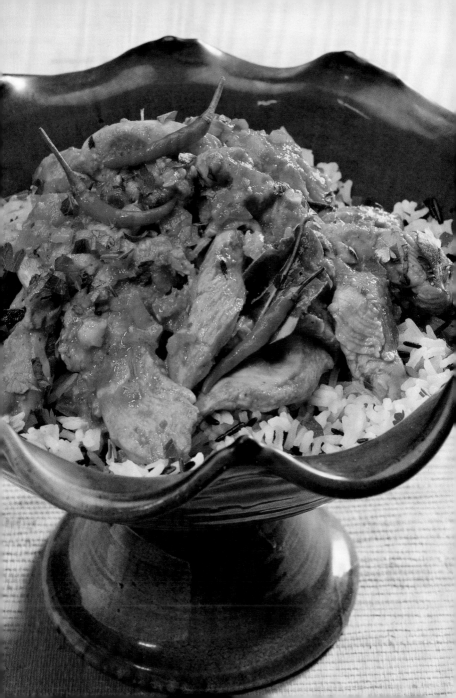

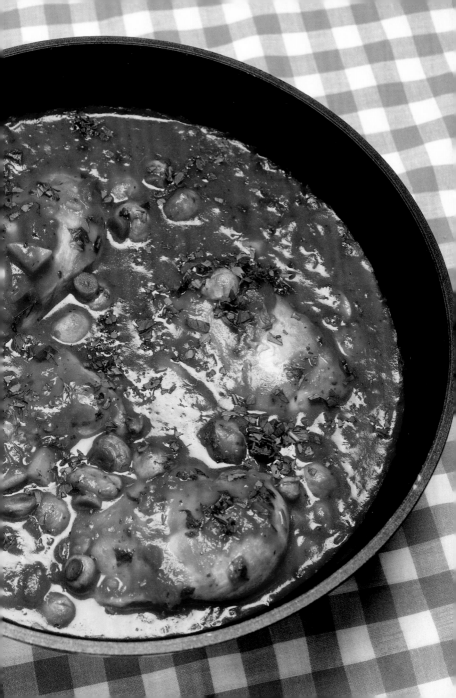

Chicken Winter Casserole

This all-in-one casserole combines chicken and vegetables in a rich tomato sauce. Fresh herbs give the sauce a real taste of Provence.

Step one Preheat the oven to 190°C/375°F/gas 5.

Step two Dry-fry the onion in a non-stick frying pan over medium heat until soft.

Step three Season the chicken on both sides and add to the pan, lightly browning on each side. Remove the chicken and place in an ovenproof dish.

Step four Add the garlic and 2 tablespoons of stock to the onion and stir in the flour. 'Cook out' for 1 minute, then add the remaining stock, the wine and tomatoes. Stir in the mixed herbs, mushrooms and swede, and bring to the boil. Pour over the chicken and cover with foil.

Step five Place in the centre of the oven for 30–35 minutes. Just before serving, sprinkle with chopped fresh parsley.

Serves 4

1 medium onion, finely chopped

4 large boneless, skinless chicken breasts

2 garlic cloves, crushed

150ml (¼ pint) chicken stock

1 tablespoon plain flour

3 tablespoons red wine

1 x 400g (14oz) tin chopped tomatoes

1 tablespoon chopped fresh mixed herbs

115g (4oz) button mushrooms

115g (4oz) swede, peeled and diced

1 tablespoon chopped fresh parsley, to garnish

salt and freshly ground black pepper

per serving:
235 kcal/8.6g fat

Coconut and Coriander Chicken

This mild creamy chicken dish is truly delicious served with rice or noodles. Chopping the coriander really finely gives the sauce a soothing, pale green colour.

Serves 4

4 boneless, skinless chicken breasts, cut into chunks

2 medium red onions, finely chopped

2 garlic cloves, crushed

150ml (¼ pint) hot vegetable stock

2 teaspoons ground coriander

1 tablespoon plain flour

1 x 400ml tin reduced-fat coconut milk

1 tablespoon chopped fresh coriander

2 tablespoons virtually fat-free fromage frais

salt and freshly ground black pepper

per serving:
282 kcal/4.3g fat

Step one Preheat a non-stick pan or wok. Season the chicken chunks with salt and black pepper and dry-fry in the pan or wok over medium heat for 6–7 minutes until they start to colour. Remove from the pan and set aside.

Step two Add the onions and garlic to the pan or wok and gently cook until soft. Add 2 tablespoons of stock and mix well. Stir in the ground coriander and the flour and 'cook out' for 1 minute.

Step three Gradually add the remaining stock and the coconut milk, stirring continuously to prevent any lumps from forming.

Step four Return the chicken to the pan and gently simmer for 10 minutes to ensure that the chicken is fully cooked. Remove from the heat, stir in the chopped coriander and the fromage frais. Serve immediately.

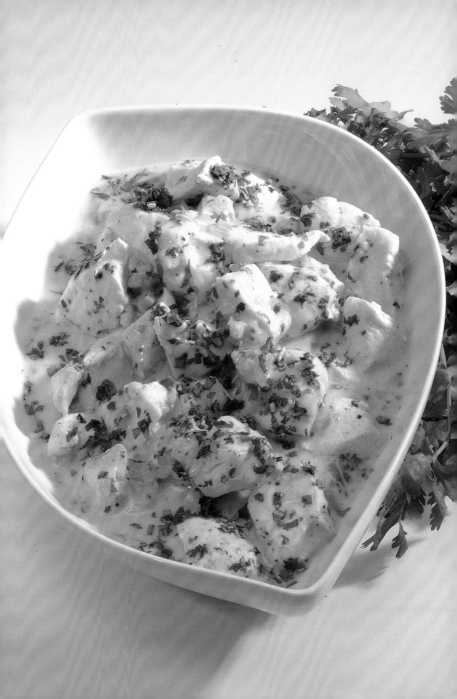

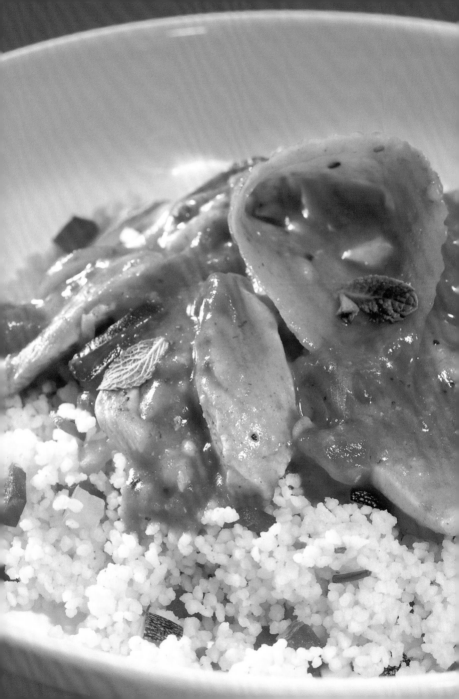

Tunisian Chicken

The rich spicy sauce in this recipe is created partly by the use of orange juice. Vegetarians can substitute Quorn or soya for the chicken.

Step one Preheat a non-stick frying pan on medium heat. Add the onion and dry-fry for 2–3 minutes until soft. Add the chicken and garlic and cook briskly, turning the chicken regularly to seal on all sides.

Step two Add the spices with 2–3 tablespoons of stock and sprinkle the flour over. Mix well, 'cooking out' the flour for 1 minute.

Step three Gradually mix in the remaining stock. Add the oregano, tomatoes, orange peel and juice. Cover and gently simmer for 20 minutes.

Step four Season to taste with salt and black pepper and serve hot with couscous or rice.

Serves 4

1 large red onion, finely sliced

4 boneless, skinless chicken breasts, cut into strips

2 garlic cloves, chopped

1 teaspoon coriander seeds

1 teaspoon ground cumin

1 teaspoon ground cinnamon

½ teaspoon cayenne pepper

6 cardamom pods, crushed with seeds removed

300ml (½ pint) chicken stock

2 tablespoons plain flour

1 tablespoon chopped fresh oregano

1 x 400g (14oz) tin chopped tomatoes

2 pieces orange peel

150ml (¼ pint) orange juice

salt and freshly ground black pepper

per serving:
280 kcal/3.8g fat

Oven-baked Chicken Tikka Masala

Oven-baked means no additional fat is required. The yoghurt adds a rich, smooth, creamy texture as well as toning down the spicy flavour.

Serves 4

4 boneless, skinless chicken breasts

600ml (1 pint) tomato Passata

300ml (½ pint) low-fat natural yoghurt

2 tablespoons chopped fresh coriander

mint leaves, to garnish

salt and freshly ground black pepper

for the tikka paste

1 small red onion

4 tablespoons tomato purée

1 teaspoon ground cumin

⅓ teaspoon ground cinnamon

1 x 2.5cm (1in) piece fresh ginger, grated

2 garlic cloves, crushed

1 small red chilli, seeded and chopped

juice of 1 lime

2 teaspoons vegetable bouillon stock powder

Step one Preheat the oven to 200°C/400°F/gas 6.

Step two Cut the chicken into chunks, place in a bowl and season well with salt and black pepper.

Step three Place the tikka paste ingredients in a food processor and blend until smooth. Spread the tikka mixture over the chicken, coating on all sides. Leave to marinate for 20 minutes.

Step four Transfer to a non-stick roasting tin and place in the oven for 15 minutes until lightly roasted. Remove from the oven and stir in the tomato Passata. Return to the oven for a further 10 minutes to heat through.

Step five Just before serving, stir in the yoghurt and chopped coriander. Spoon into a warmed serving dish and garnish with mint leaves.

per serving:
334 kcal/9.6g fat

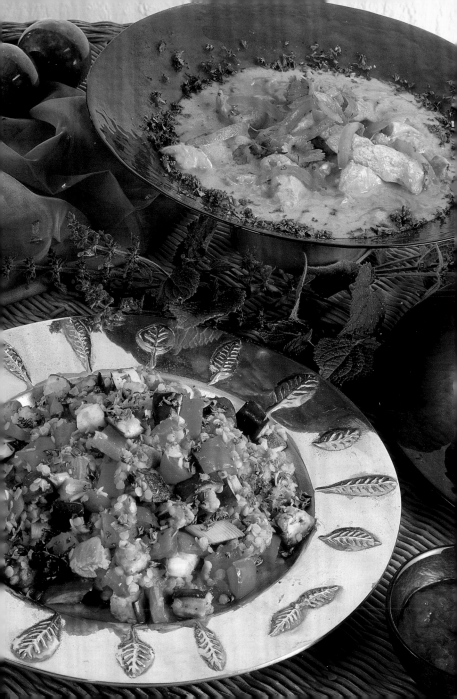

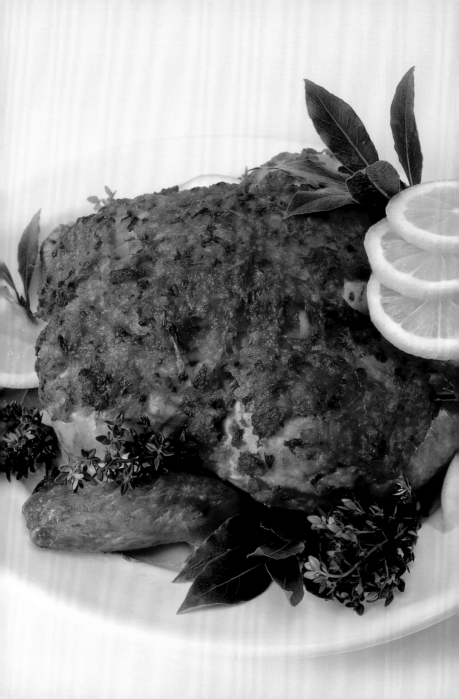

Lemon Roast Chicken with Fresh Herb Stuffing

Simple roast chicken can be enjoyed by everyone – just remember to remove the skin. Breast meat is much leaner than the leg or thigh, as the fat drips down through the bird as it cooks. Try to drain as much fat as possible from the cooking juices when making the accompanying gravy.

Step one Preheat the oven to 180°C/350°F/gas 4.

Step two Prepare the chicken by washing it well inside and out. Remove as much skin as possible from the chicken and season with salt and black pepper.

Step three Place a non-stick pan over medium heat. When it is hot, add the onion and garlic and dry-fry for 4–5 minutes until soft. Add the breadcrumbs and herbs with a little black pepper. Mix in the 300ml (½ pint) hot stock and 1 teaspoon of lemon zest, then remove from the heat and allow to cool.

Step four Once it has cooled, spoon the stuffing into the chicken's neck cavity (the smaller of the two cavities), and press in well. Press the remaining stuffing onto the chicken, covering the outside. Push one lemon inside the other cavity. Squeeze the juice from the remaining lemon and pour over the chicken.

Step five Place the chicken on a rack over a non-stick roasting tin, cover with foil and place in the oven for 1–1½ hours, depending on the size of the chicken (allow 30 minutes per 450g/1lb, plus an extra 30 minutes).

Step six Once it's cooked, remove the chicken from the roasting tin and wrap with foil to keep hot. Rinse out the tin with 600ml (1 pint) chicken stock and pour through a sieve into a gravy separator. Drain off the juices, and heat in a pan. Thicken with gravy powder.

Serves 4

1 medium free-range or organic chicken (approx. 1.5kg/3lb)

1 medium onion, finely chopped

2 garlic cloves, crushed

115g (4oz) fresh breadcrumbs

1 tablespoon each chopped fresh thyme and parsley

2 teaspoons chopped fresh rosemary

300ml (½ pint) hot chicken stock

2 lemons

salt and freshly ground black pepper

for the gravy

600ml (1 pint) chicken stock, for the gravy

1 tablespoon gravy powder

per serving:

425 kcal/13g fat

Turkey and Pepper Stroganoff

Stroganoff, as the name suggests, is a dish that originated in Russia. This modern variation, using lean turkey instead of beef, tastes and looks vibrant, but is not as high in fat as the original.

Serves 4

450g (1lb) lean cooked turkey meat, cut into strips

1 medium onion, chopped

1 red pepper, seeded and diced

2 garlic cloves, crushed

300ml (½ pint) chicken stock

1 tablespoon plain flour

150ml (¼ pint) Madeira wine

225g (8oz) small chestnut mushrooms, sliced

2 teaspoons Dijon mustard

300ml (½ pint) virtually fat-free fromage frais

2 tablespoons chopped fresh parsley

paprika, to dust

4 lemon wedges, to garnish

salt and freshly ground black pepper

per serving:
280 kcal/3.4g fat

Step one Preheat a non-stick frying pan or wok over medium heat. Spray with a little olive oil to coat the pan and add the cooked turkey and the onion. Dry-fry for 2–3 minutes until the onion starts to soften.

Step two Add the red pepper and garlic and cook for a further minute. Add 2–3 tablespoons of the stock and sprinkle the flour over. Mix well with a wooden spoon and 'cook out' the flour for 1 minute.

Step three Add the remaining stock and the Madeira wine, stirring continuously, followed by the mushrooms. Stir in the mustard and cook for a further 2–3 minutes. Remove the pan from the heat and stir in the fromage frais and parsley.

Step four Check the seasoning, dust with paprika and garnish with lemon wedges.

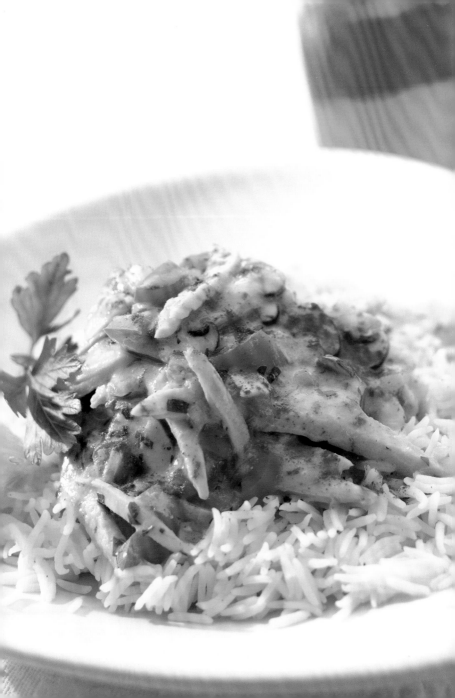

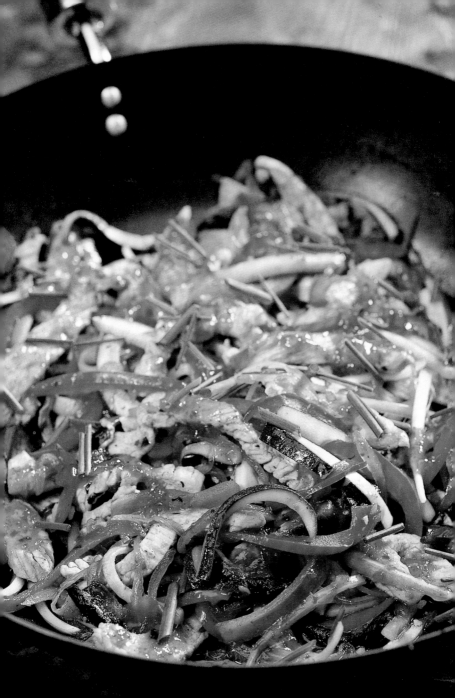

Turkey and Ginger Stir-fry

This recipe is ideal for using up any oddments of vegetables you have to hand. You can substitute leeks or root vegetables such as thinly sliced carrots or parsnips for the red pepper, courgettes and mushrooms, but they may need slightly longer cooking times.

Step one Heat a non-stick wok or frying pan over medium heat, add the turkey strips and dry-fry for 5–6 minutes or until just cooked. Remove from the pan and set aside.

Step two Return the pan to the heat and add the onion, red pepper and courgettes and dry-fry for 2–3 minutes. Add the mushrooms and ginger, mixing well. Return the turkey to the pan and continue cooking.

Step three Mix together the soy sauce, honey (or chutney) and chilli and add to the pan, coating the meat and vegetables. Stir-fry, combining all the ingredients, until the meat is fully cooked.

Step four Serve immediately, heaped on a bed of noodles or instant rice.

Serves 4

450g (1lb) turkey fillets, cut into strips

1 medium red onion, finely sliced

1 red pepper, seeded and sliced

2 small courgettes, sliced

115g (4oz) chestnut mushrooms, sliced

2 teaspoons fresh ginger, finely chopped

1 tablespoon light soy sauce

1 tablespoon clear honey or mango chutney

2 teaspoons chilli sauce

per serving:

229 kcal/2.4g fat

Breast of Pheasant with Wild Mushrooms

Use fresh pheasant, if in season, or frozen. If you have difficulty finding wild mushrooms, use open-cup cultivated ones instead.

Serves 4

2 pheasants, breasts and fillets removed and carcase washed

2 medium onions, sliced

2 medium carrots, sliced

1 small leek, trimmed and sliced

1 celery stick, trimmed and sliced

350g (12oz) wild mushrooms, diced

300ml (½ pint) white wine

1 large garlic clove, crushed

1 tablespoon fresh white breadcrumbs

1 tablespoon chopped fresh parsley

2 tablespoons brandy

salt and freshly ground black pepper

to garnish

1 orange, sliced (optional)

small bunch watercress

per serving:

405 kcal/10.6g fat

Step one Put the carcase in a large pan. Add half the sliced onions and carrots, cover with water and bring to the boil. Cover and gently simmer for 2 hours. Strain the stock into a pan and discard the vegetables and carcase. Boil the stock rapidly to reduce to about 150ml (¼ pint) and reserve.

Step two Place the leek, celery and remaining onions and carrots in a pan with a little water. Season lightly and simmer until just tender. Drain and add the cooking liquor to the stock. Reserve the vegetables. Preheat the oven to 200°C/400°F/gas 6.

Step three Season the mushrooms lightly. Place them in a pan over medium heat and add the wine. Cook for 10–12 minutes. Drain, reserving the cooking liquor. Finely chop about 75g (3oz) of the mushrooms.

Step four To make the stuffing, cut the fillets into small pieces. Add to a food processor with the garlic and work until finely chopped. Place in a bowl and mix in the breadcrumbs, parsley, 1 tablespoon of brandy and chopped mushrooms. Set aside.

Step five Cut a slit in each pheasant breast to make a pocket and divide stuffing between each pocket. Press the edges of each slit together and place the breasts in an ovenproof dish.

Step six Make the sauce by adding the cooked vegetables, the reduced stock and all the cooking liquor to a liquidiser. Blend until smooth, then transfer to a pan on medium heat, adding the remaining mushrooms and 1 tablespoon of brandy. Warm through, then pour the sauce over the pheasant breasts and cook in the oven for 30–40 minutes, depending on their size.

Step seven Garnish the dish with the watercress and orange slices (if using) and serve with a selection of vegetables.

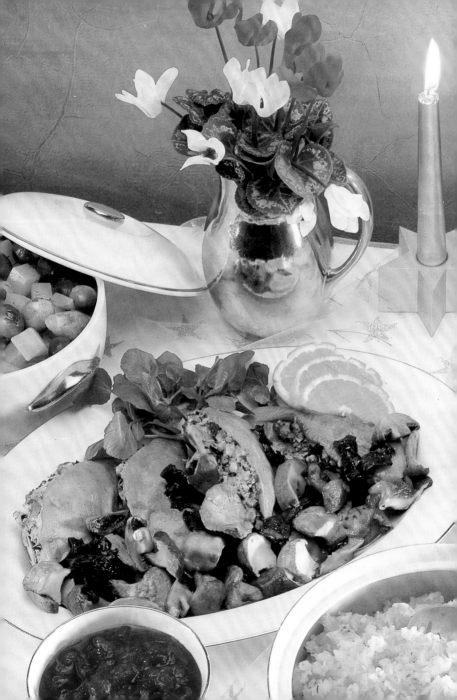

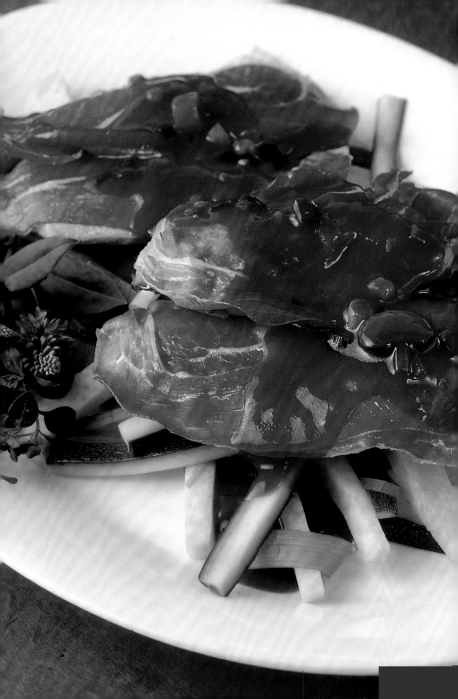

Pheasant Wrapped in Parma Ham with Red Wine

Pheasant has a much stronger flavour than most poultry, although the breast meat has a much lighter flavour than that of the dark leg meat.

Step one Season the pheasant breasts on both sides with plenty of black pepper, then wrap each breast in a slice of Parma ham.

Step two Preheat a non-stick pan over medium heat. Add the pheasant and dry-fry on both sides for 5–6 minutes until lightly browned. Remove from the pan and place on a plate.

Step three Add the onion to the pan and gently cook until lightly coloured. Add the celery and 2 tablespoons of stock. Sprinkle the flour over and 'cook out' for 1 minute. Slowly stir in the remaining stock, along with the mushrooms and wine.

Step four Return the pheasant to the pan and add the herbs. Gently simmer for 15–20 minutes until the sauce has reduced and the pheasant is cooked through. Serve with seasonal vegetables.

Serves 4

4 skinless pheasant breasts (approx. 115g/4oz each)

freshly ground black pepper

4 lean slices Parma ham

1 medium red onion, finely chopped

2 celery sticks, finely chopped

1 chicken stock cube dissolved in 300ml (½ pint) water

1 tablespoon plain flour

225g (8oz) chestnut mushrooms, sliced

1 wine glass red wine

2 tablespoons chopped fresh mixed herbs

per serving:
350 kcal/15g fat

Lemon-baked Guinea Fowl

Guinea fowl is a light-flavoured game bird. It is not as strong in flavour as pheasant but is stronger than chicken.

Serves 4

3 baby leeks, finely chopped

4 skinless guinea fowl breasts

300ml (½ pint) skimmed milk

2 teaspoons vegetable bouillon stock powder

150ml (¼ pint) dry white wine

1 tablespoon cornflour

zest and juice of 1 lemon

1 tablespoon chopped fresh parsley, to garnish

salt and freshly ground black pepper

per serving:

278 kcal/4.2g fat

Step one Preheat the oven to 180°C/350°F/gas 4.

Step two Preheat a non-stick pan over medium heat, then add the leeks and dry-fry until soft. Place in the base of an ovenproof dish.

Step three Season the guinea fowl breasts on both sides with salt and black pepper and add to the pan, browning them on both sides. Transfer to the ovenproof dish and place on top of the leeks.

Step four Meanwhile, heat the milk, stock powder and wine in a pan over medium heat. Slake the cornflour with a little cold milk and stir into the pan. Reduce the heat and simmer for 2–3 minutes; as the sauce thickens, add the lemon zest and juice. Pour the sauce over the guinea fowl and cover with foil.

Step five Bake for 20 minutes until fully cooked through.

Step six Transfer to a serving dish and sprinkle with the chopped parsley. Serve with a selection of green vegetables and potatoes.

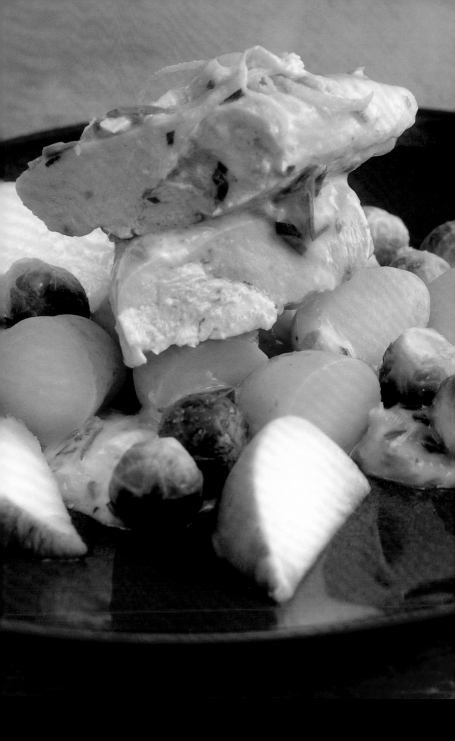

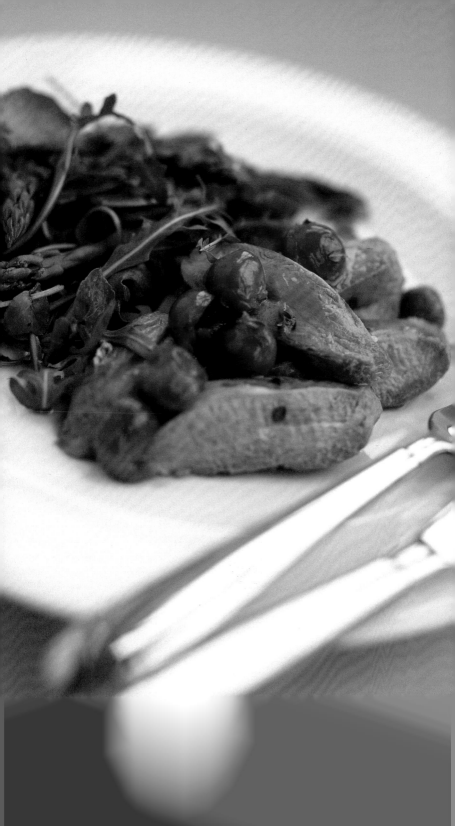

Low-fat Duck with Black Cherries

A delicate fruity sauce rounds off this exotic dish. Duck meat without the fatty skin is very lean.

Step one Preheat the oven to 200°C/400°F/gas 6.

Step two Prepare the duck by removing all the skin with a sharp knife. Season each breast well with salt and black pepper. With the sharp knife, slash the duck several times and place in an ovenproof dish.

Step three Heat the cherries, thyme and orange juice in a pan. Mix the arrowroot with a little cold water to a paste and stir into the sauce. Simmer until thickened, then pour the sauce over the duck. Place in the oven for 10–12 minutes.

Step four Remove the duck from the oven and allow to rest for 5 minutes.

Step five Strain the juices from the roasting dish into the sauce and stir in the chopped mint. Carve the duck into pieces and serve with the hot cherry sauce and some green vegetables.

Serves 4

4 x 175g (6oz)
duck breasts

salt and freshly
ground black pepper

for the sauce

275g (10oz) jar
morello cherries

few sprigs fresh thyme

150ml (¼ pint)
orange juice

2 teaspoons arrowroot

chopped fresh
mint leaves

per serving:

468 kcal/4.7g fat

For a video masterclass on knife skills, go to
www.mykitchentable.co.uk/videos/knifeskills

Cottage Pie with Leek and Potato Topping

This recipe also works well using minced lamb or pork instead of beef.

Serves 4

450g (1lb) lean minced beef

1 onion, chopped

2 carrots, chopped

2 tablespoons plain flour

300ml (½ pint) stock

1 tablespoon tomato purée

1 tablespoon mixed dried herbs

for the topping

675g (1½ lb) potatoes, peeled and chopped

2 leeks, trimmed and sliced

2 tablespoons skimmed milk

50g (2oz) low-fat Cheddar, grated (optional)

salt and freshly ground black pepper

per serving:
with cheese:

359 kcal/8g fat

without cheese:

327 kcal/6.2g fat

Step one Preheat the oven to 190°C/375°F/gas 5.

Step two Boil the potatoes until soft, adding the leeks 5 minutes before the end of cooking.

Step three Meanwhile, dry-fry the beef for 3–4 minutes in a non-stick frying pan over medium heat. Remove from the pan and strain. Discard the liquid and put the meat to one side. Wipe out the pan. Return the meat to the pan.

Step four Add the onion and carrots and stir in the flour. Gradually add the stock, tomato purée and dried herbs. Bring to the boil and stir until thickened. Season with salt and black pepper. Transfer to an ovenproof dish.

Step five Drain the potatoes and leeks and mash with a little milk and half the Cheddar (if using). Season to taste with salt and black pepper. Place on top of the beef mixture. Sprinkle with the remaining Cheddar (if using). Bake for 25 minutes until golden.

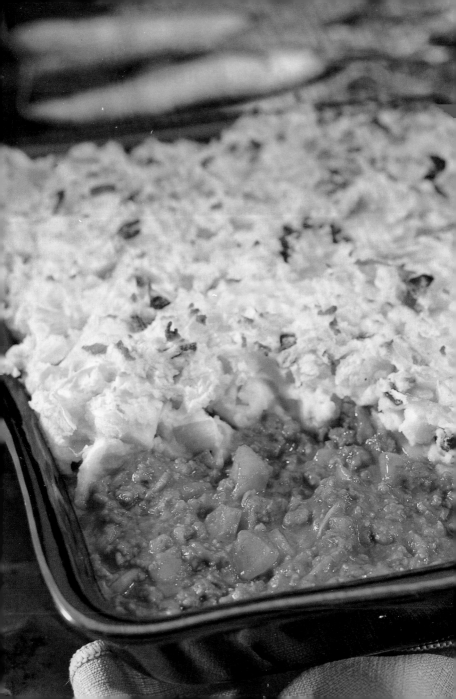

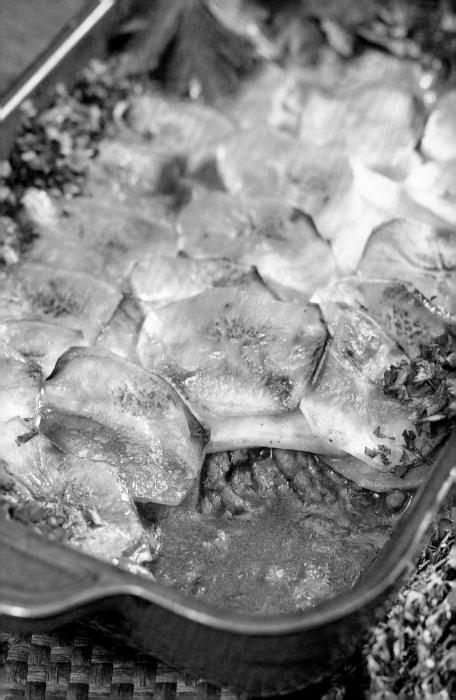

Minced Beef and Potato Pie

To make a richer sauce, you could substitute some of the beef stock with stout or real ale, but this will increase the calories!

Step one Preheat the oven to 190°C/375°F/gas 5.

Step two Preheat a non-stick frying pan. Add the minced beef and dry-fry over medium heat until it changes colour. Strain through a metal sieve to remove as much fat as possible, then wipe out the pan with kitchen paper.

Step three Add the onions and garlic to the pan and dry-fry for 2–3 minutes until soft. Add the thyme and return the beef to the pan. Add 2 tablespoons of stock and sprinkle the flour on top.

Step four Mix well, cooking over a low heat for 1 minute, then gradually add the remaining stock. Gently simmer for 10 minutes to allow the mixture to thicken, stirring occasionally. Add a little gravy browning for colour if desired and transfer to an ovenproof dish.

Step five Cover with slices of potato and brush with the soy sauce. Season well with black pepper and place in the oven for 30–35 minutes until the potatoes are cooked and golden brown.

Step six Sprinkle with chopped parsley and serve with a selection of fresh vegetables.

Serves 4

450g (1lb) lean minced beef

2 onions, finely chopped

1 garlic clove, crushed

2 teaspoons chopped fresh thyme

600ml (1 pint) beef stock

2 tablespoons plain flour

a little gravy browning (optional)

4 large potatoes, thinly sliced

1 tablespoon light soy sauce

freshly ground black pepper

1 tablespoon chopped fresh parsley, to garnish

per serving:

409 kcal/11.8g fat

Boeuf à la Bourguignonne

This modern version of the renowned French dish does not contain the traditional bacon lardons. It is lighter in fat but still meltingly delicious.

Serves 6

1kg (2¼lb) lean braising beef

2 medium onions, finely chopped

2 garlic cloves, crushed

2 teaspoons chopped fresh thyme

2 beef stock cubes dissolved in 300ml (½ pint) water

2 tablespoons plain flour

1 bottle red wine

300ml (½ pint) tomato Passata

4 large carrots

3 celery sticks, cut into 5cm (2in) batons

175g (6oz) button mushrooms

20 baby onions, peeled

bouquet garni

chopped fresh parsley, to garnish

salt and freshly ground black pepper

Step one Preheat the oven to 180°C/350°F/gas 4.

Step two Cut the beef into 2.5cm (1in) dice, removing all fat and sinew. Season with salt and black pepper. Preheat a small pan on medium heat and add the diced beef. Seal the beef on all sides in small batches until lightly browned. Remove from the pan and set aside.

Step three Add the onions, garlic and thyme to the pan and gently cook over medium heat for 2–3 minutes until soft. Add 2 tablespoons of the stock, then sprinkle the flour over, stir well and cook for a further minute to 'cook out' the flour. Slowly stir in the remaining stock, along with the wine and tomato Passata.

Step four Cut the carrots into 4cm (1½in) lengths. Using a small, sharp knife, carefully peel away the outside skins to form the carrot pieces into barrel shapes. Add the carrots, along with the celery, mushrooms and baby onions, to the sauce.

Step five Place the beef in the bottom of a large casserole dish and pour the sauce and the vegetables over. Add the bouquet garni and cover with a lid. Place in the oven for 35–40 minutes until the sauce has reduced.

Step six Remove the bouquet garni and garnish with parsley before serving.

per serving:
500 kcal/15g fat

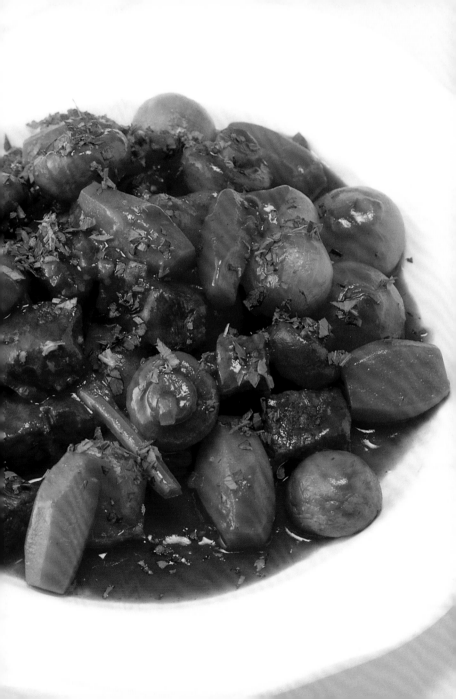

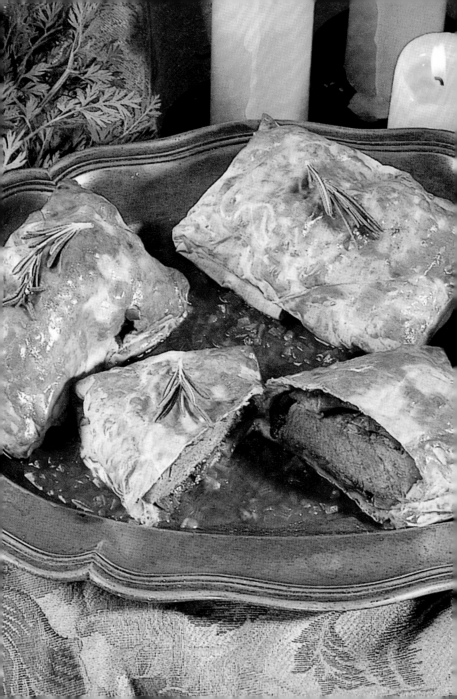

Beef Wellingtons with Red Wine Sauce

This simplified Beef Wellington recipe reduces the fat and calorie content considerably. The individual Wellingtons can be made in advance, covered with a damp cloth and stored in the refrigerator.

Step one Preheat the oven to 200°C/400°F/gas 6. Seal the steaks on both sides in a hot non-stick pan, seasoning well. Remove from the pan and set aside, reserving the pan for later.

Step two Place the wild mushrooms in a small pan with the stock, garlic and thyme. Cook over a low heat and gently simmer for 15–20 minutes until soft.

Step three In a non-stick frying pan, dry-fry the onion over medium heat until it just starts to colour. Add the mushrooms and stock and the parsley and continue to cook until all the liquid has reduced to a paste. Allow to cool.

Step four Take a sheet of filo pastry and brush with the beaten egg. Fold the sheet in half, place a teaspoon of the mushroom mixture in the centre, sit a steak on top and spread with another teaspoon of the mushroom mixture. Fold the pastry around the beef, enclosing it in a tight parcel. Trim any excess pastry with scissors. Repeat with the remaining steaks.

Step five Place the parcels on a non-stick baking sheet and brush with beaten egg. Bake for 12–20 minutes, according to your preference.

Step six Meanwhile, make the sauce by dry-frying the shallots over medium heat in the meat pan until soft. Add 1 tablespoon of stock and sprinkle the flour over. Mix well and cook for 1–2 minutes to 'cook out' the flour, then gradually stir in the remaining stock and the wine. Gently simmer for 10 minutes until thickened, adding a drop of gravy browning for colour.

Step seven Serve the Wellingtons straight from the oven with a selection of vegetables and the accompanying sauce.

Serves 4

4 x 175g (6oz) fillet steaks, trimmed of fat and cut into 4 equal-sized steaks

25g (1oz) dried, mixed wild forest mushrooms

150ml (¼ pint) beef stock

2 garlic cloves, crushed

1 teaspoon finely chopped fresh thyme

1 medium onion, finely chopped

1 tablespoon chopped fresh parsley

4 sheets filo pastry

1 egg, beaten with 2 tablespoons milk

salt and freshly ground black pepper

for the sauce

2 small shallots, finely chopped

150ml (¼ pint) beef stock

2 teaspoons plain flour

300ml (½ pint) red wine

gravy browning

per serving:
348 kcal/12.7g fat

Rich Spaghetti Bolognese

This classic Italian dish consists of lean minced beef in a rich, herby sauce. Traditionally, the beef and onions are fried in olive oil. In this low-fat version, we dry-fry the minced beef to release the fat. Adding the sun-dried tomatoes gives a strong, robust flavour, but ensure you use the dried ones in packets, since the ones in jars contain oil.

Serves 4

450g (1lb) lean minced beef

2 garlic cloves, crushed

1 large onion, finely diced

2 medium carrots, finely diced

2 beef stock cubes

2 x 400g (14oz) tins chopped tomatoes

2 tablespoons tomato purée

1 tablespoon chopped fresh mixed herbs (oregano, marjoram, basil, parsley)

8 sun-dried tomatoes, finely chopped

225g (8oz) spaghetti

chopped fresh herbs, to garnish

salt and freshly ground black pepper

Step one Dry-fry the minced beef in a non-stick pan over medium heat until it starts to change colour. Remove the beef from the pan and wipe out the pan with kitchen paper. Return the meat to the pan, add the garlic and onion and continue cooking over medium heat for a further 2–3 minutes, stirring the ingredients well.

Step two Add the carrots, stock cubes, tinned tomatoes, tomato purée, herbs and sun-dried tomatoes and mix well to allow the stock cubes to dissolve. Reduce the heat to a gentle simmer, season to taste with salt and black pepper, cover with a lid, and continue to cook for 30 minutes until the sauce thickens.

Step three Meanwhile, bring a large pan of salted water to the boil. Add the spaghetti and cook for 20–25 minutes until the spaghetti is soft but slightly firm in the centre. Drain through a colander.

Step four Arrange the spaghetti on warmed serving plates and pour the sauce on top. Garnish with chopped fresh herbs.

per serving:

521 kcal/12.8g fat

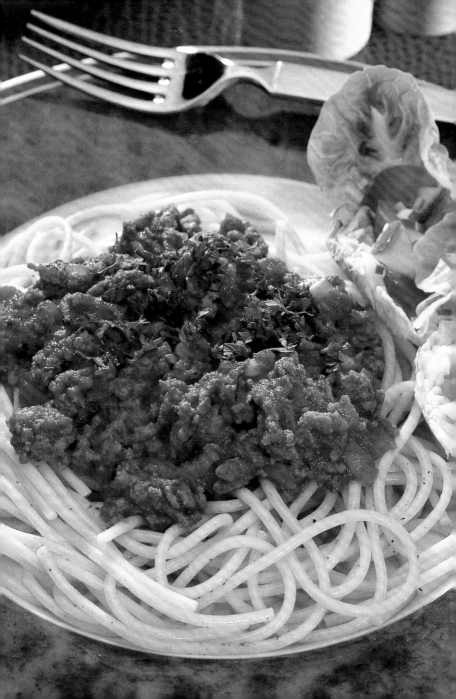

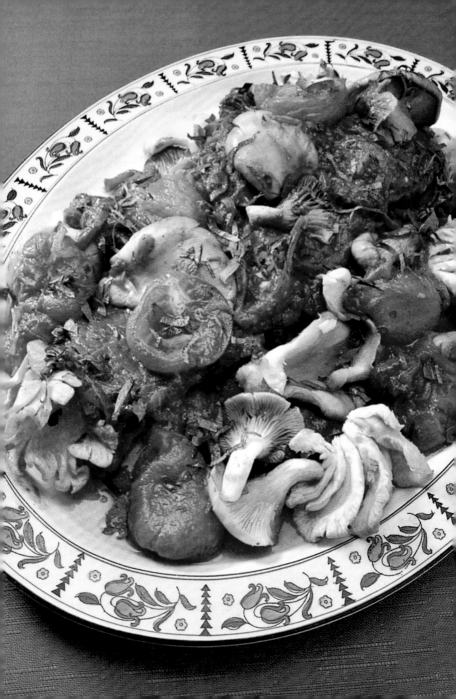

Tomato-braised Beef with Oyster Mushrooms

In this recipe, ripe tomatoes form the base of the rich sauce. For a lighter sauce, you could use beef stock instead of wine.

Step one Preheat the oven to 180°C/350°F/gas 4.

Step two Preheat a non-stick frying pan over medium-high heat. Season the meat well with salt and black pepper. Add it to the pan and dry-fry until browned on both sides. Transfer to a flameproof casserole.

Step three Add the onions to the pan and soften for 3–4 minutes over medium heat. Sprinkle the thyme over the onions and then add the wine and stock cube. Stir well.

Step four Scatter the tomatoes over the beef and then pour the onion and wine mixture over. Cover and cook in the oven for 35 minutes.

Step five Remove the beef from the oven and add the mushrooms and the tomato purée. Cover and return to the oven for a further 25 minutes or until the beef is tender.

Step six Just before serving, sprinkle with chopped fresh coriander. Serve with potatoes and unlimited vegetables.

Serves 6

900g (2lb) lean rump or braising steak

2 red onions, finely sliced

2 teaspoons chopped fresh thyme

300ml (½ pint) red wine

½ beef stock cube

450g (1lb) fresh plum tomatoes, skinned and halved

350g (12oz) oyster mushrooms

2 tablespoons tomato purée

chopped fresh coriander, to garnish

salt and freshly ground black pepper

per serving:
264 kcal/9g fat

Roast Beef with Yorkshire Pudding, Dry-roast Potatoes and Parsnips

All the flavour of a traditional Sunday roast without all the fat and calories.

Serves 6

1kg (2¼lb) joint lean beef, topside

1 onion, finely diced

1 carrot, diced

1 celery stick, diced

2 teaspoons mixed dried herbs

600ml (1 pint) beef stock

1 tablespoon cornflour

1–2 drops gravy browning

for the dry-roast potatoes and parsnips

450g (1lb) potatoes, peeled and cut in half

8 parsnips, peeled

1 tablespoon soy sauce, diluted in 2 tablespoons of water (optional)

for the Yorkshire pudding batter

115g (4oz) plain flour

1 egg

pinch of salt

150ml (¼ pint) skimmed milk

per serving:

beef: 218 kcal/8.3g fat;
dry-roast potatoes and parsnips:
106 kcal/0.9g fat;
Yorkshire pudding:
79 kcal/1.3g fat

Step one Preheat the oven to 180°C/350°F/gas 4. Remove as much fat as possible from the beef.

Step two Put the onion, carrot, celery and herbs in a roasting tin or ovenproof dish. Sit the beef on top and pour 300ml (½ pint) water around it. Place in the oven. Allow 15 minutes per 450g (lb) plus 15 minutes for rare beef, 20 minutes per 450g (1lb) plus 20 minutes for medium rare, and 25 minutes per 450g (1lb) plus 30 minutes if you like your beef well done.

Step three Cook the potatoes and parsnips separately in boiling water. Drain and place in a non-stick roasting tin. Roast in the top of the oven for 35–40 minutes until golden brown. You can baste the vegetables with the diluted soy sauce if they appear to dry out, depending on your oven.

Step four Forty minutes before the beef is ready, make the Yorkshire pudding batter by blending the flour with the egg, a pinch of salt and a little milk to a smooth paste. Whisk in the remaining milk until smooth. Preheat a six-mould non-stick Yorkshire pudding tin for 2 minutes in the oven. Remove and half-fill each mould with batter. Return to the oven and increase the heat to 200°C/400°F/gas 6 for 35–40 minutes.

Step five When the beef is cooked, remove it from the tin and wrap in foil to keep warm. Allow the beef to rest for 5–10 minutes. Meanwhile, place the roasting tin over medium heat and add the beef stock to the tin juices. Slake the cornflour with a little water and add to the tin. Stir well as the gravy thickens. Add gravy browning as required.

Step six Carve the beef and serve with the Yorkshire pudding, potatoes and parsnips, gravy and seasonal vegetables.

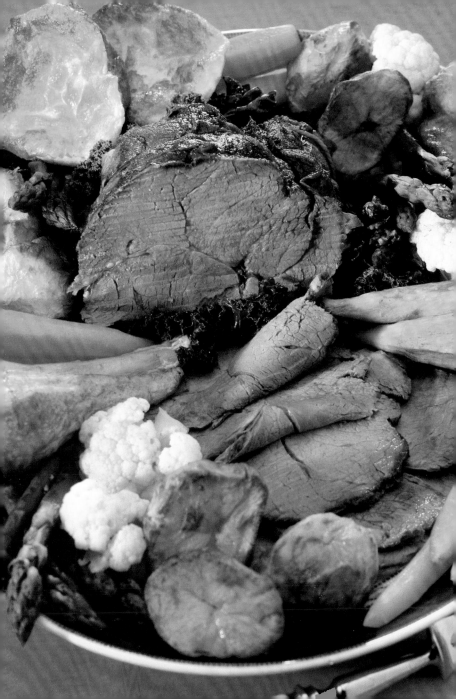

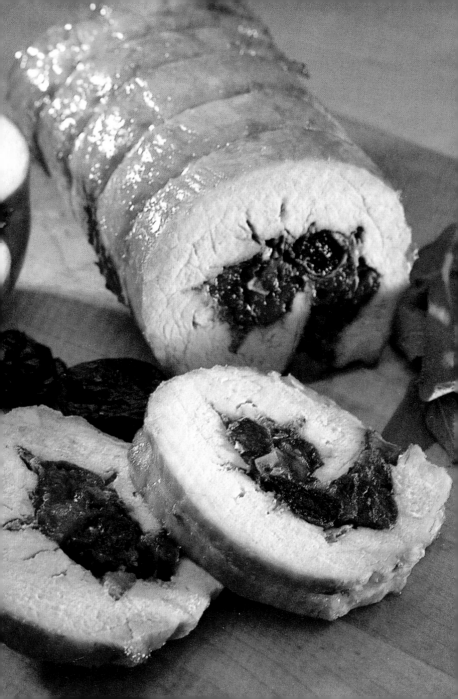

Honey-roast Pork with Prune and Apple Stuffing

This version of pork with apples and prunes, slowly roasting in the oven, will evoke the flavours and aroma of Normandy – a healthy taste of France.

Step one Preheat the oven to 200°C/400°F/gas 6.

Step two Trim all the fat from the pork, then weigh the meat to calculate the cooking time: you need to allow 30 minutes per 450g (1lb), plus 30 minutes. Place the pork on a chopping board and season well with salt and black pepper.

Step three Dry-fry the onion in a non-stick pan over medium heat until soft. Add the prunes, apple, sage and 150ml (¼ pint) of the stock. Cook briskly for 1–2 minutes, then allow to cool.

Step four Spread three-quarters of the prune and apple mixture on the pork. Roll the pork up and tie with string. Place the pork in a roasting tin. Spoon the honey over the pork and pour 300ml (½ pint) of water around the meat. Cover with foil and cook in the oven.

Step five Make the sauce by placing the remaining prune mixture in a pan. Add the wine and remaining stock and bring to the boil. Blend the cornflour with a little water and use to thicken the sauce. For a smooth sauce, place in a liquidiser and blend until smooth.

Step six Serve the pork with the sauce and accompany with potatoes and fresh vegetables.

Serves 6

1.5kg (3lb) lean boned pork loin

1 medium onion, finely chopped

225g (8oz) 'no soak' prunes, stoned

1 cooking apple, peeled and grated

2 tablespoons chopped fresh sage

600ml (1 pint) vegetable stock

3 tablespoons clear honey

1 wine glass red wine

1 tablespoon cornflour

salt and freshly ground black pepper

per serving:
441 kcal/8.2g fat

Gammon with Pineapple Rice

Gammon and pineapple are a long-standing partnership. This colourful, easy recipe updates the combination and introduces healthy brown rice.

Serves 1

1 gammon steak

1 small onion, finely chopped

1 small tin pineapple chunks in natural juice

½ vegetable stock cube

50g (2oz) brown rice

50g (2oz) tinned or frozen peas

½ red pepper, seeded and sliced

dash of soy sauce

1 tablespoon snipped fresh chives

salt and freshly ground black pepper

per serving:

431 kcal/5.5g fat

Step one Cut the gammon steak into cubes and gently dry-fry with the onion in a non-stick pan over medium heat.

Step two Add the pineapple and juice, the stock cube, rice and approximately 300ml (½ pint) water and bring to the boil. Cover and cook for 10 minutes or until the rice is tender and most of the liquid is absorbed. Add more boiling water during cooking if necessary.

Step three Stir in the peas, red pepper and soy sauce and season to taste with salt and black pepper. Finally, stir in the chives, heat through and serve immediately.

Have you made this recipe? Tell us what you think at
www.mykitchentable.co.uk/blog

96

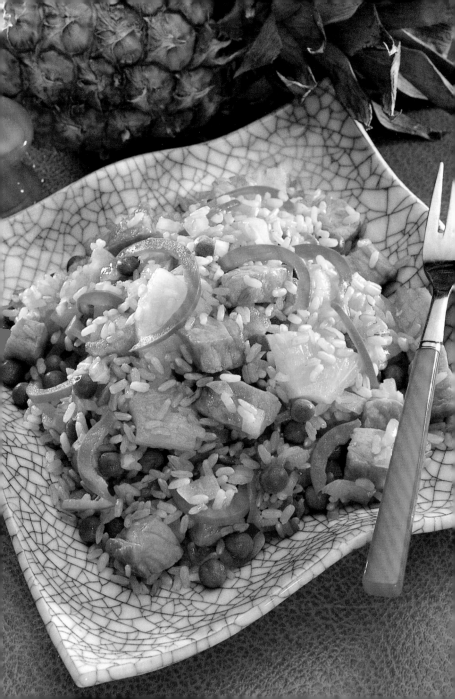

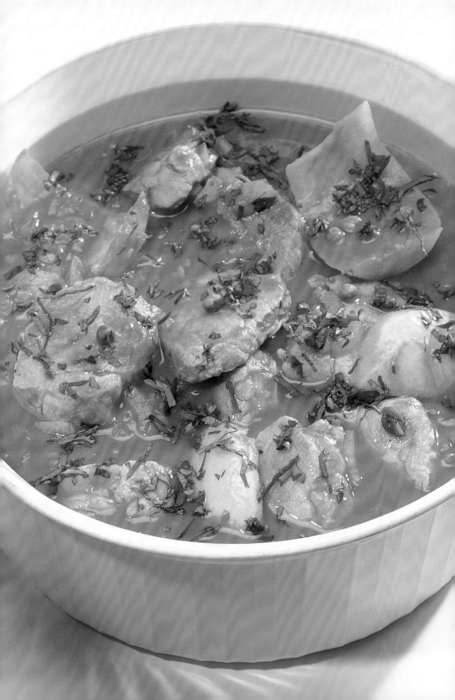

Lemon Pork with Capers

A succulent pork dish that combines unusual flavours. This recipe also works with chicken or turkey steaks.

Step one Preheat the oven to 200°C/400°F/gas 6. Preheat a non-stick frying pan or wok to a high heat.

Step two Cut the pork into chunky discs and season well with salt and black pepper. Pan-fry each piece over the high heat, to seal the meat, and place in an ovenproof dish.

Step three Reduce the heat to medium and add the onions, garlic and celery to the pan and soften. Add 2–3 tablespoons of stock to the pan, then sprinkle the flour over. Mix well, and 'cook out' the flour for 1 minute.

Step four Gradually stir in the remaining stock and add the remaining ingredients, except the parsley. Bring the sauce to the boil to allow it to thicken, then pour it over the pork. Cover with foil and place in the centre of the oven for 30–35 minutes.

Step five Remove from the oven and sprinkle over the parsley. Serve with a selection of fresh vegetables.

Serves 4

1kg (2lb) pork fillet

2 red onions, finely chopped

2 garlic cloves, crushed

2 small celery sticks, sliced

300ml (½ pint) vegetable stock

1 tablespoon plain flour

2 teaspoons chopped fresh lemon thyme

1 cinnamon stick

2–3 pieces lemon peel

1 litre (1¾ pints) tomato Passata

½ wine glass dry white wine

115g (4oz) capers

2 tablespoons chopped, fresh flat-leaf parsley, to garnish

salt and freshly ground black pepper

per serving:
473 kcal/9.7g fat

Sage and Onion Roast Pork

Spring onions form the centre to this traditional roast. Using fresh sage gives a much stronger flavour than using dried, adding depth and a distinctive herb flavour to the finished sauce.

Serves 4

1.5kg (3lb) lean pork loin joint, boned

2 onions, finely chopped

1 large cooking apple, peeled and grated

2 tablespoons chopped fresh sage

12 thin spring onions

3 tablespoons clear honey

600ml (1 pint) vegetable stock

1 tablespoon cornflour

1 wine glass white wine

salt and freshly ground black pepper

per serving:

559 kcal/14g fat

Step one Preheat the oven to 200°C/400°F/gas 6.

Step two Trim away all the fat from the pork, then weigh the joint to calculate the cooking time: allow 30 minutes per 450g (1lb), plus 30 minutes. Lay the meat out flat on a chopping board and season well with salt and black pepper.

Step three Dry-fry the onion in a non-stick pan over medium heat until soft. Add the apple and sage, stir well, then remove from the heat and allow to cool.

Step four Spread the mixture on the pork, then lay the spring onions across. Roll the pork up and tie with string. Place in a roasting tin and spoon the honey over and pour 300ml (½ pint) of the stock around the meat. Cover with foil and cook in the oven for the calculated time.

Step five Remove the pork from the tin and allow to rest, keeping it covered with foil.

Step six Add the remaining stock and the wine to the hot tin and stir well, picking up the meat juices from the bottom. Pour the mixture into a pan set over medium heat. Slake the cornflour with a little cold water and stir into the gravy. Gently simmer gently to allow the gravy to thicken.

Step seven Slice the pork and arrange on a serving dish with the accompanying sauce. Serve with potatoes, seasonal vegetables and apple sauce.

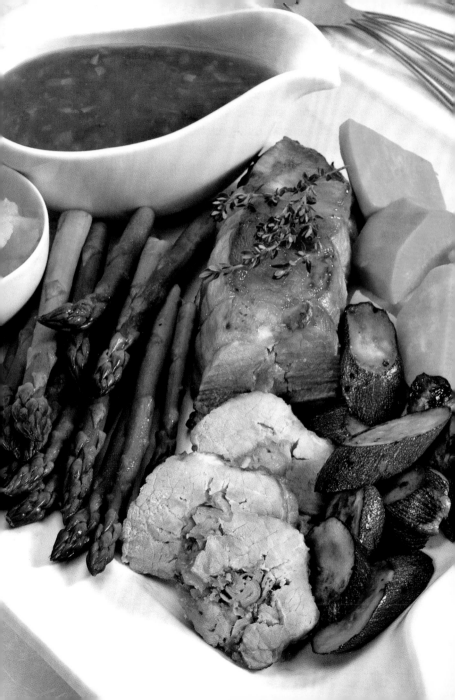

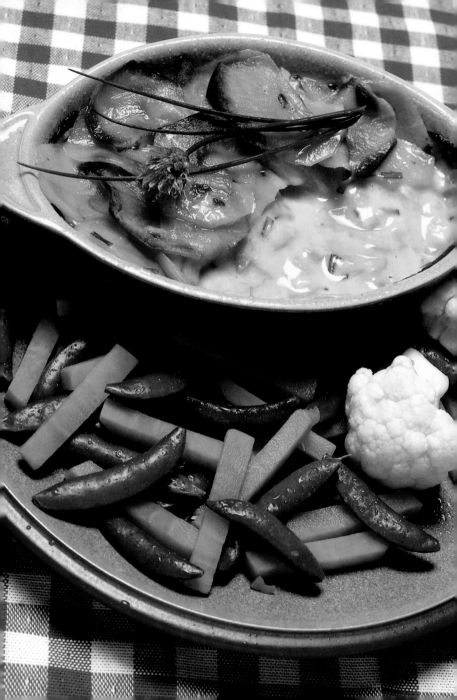

Smoked Ham and Mushroom Coddle

Coddle refers to an old recipe that uses potatoes to cover the main dish, which is then cooked in the oven. This recipe uses a creamy, low-fat ham and mushroom mixture. For a vegetarian version, replace the ham with a selection of frozen vegetables or tinned beans.

Step one Preheat the oven to 190°C/ 375°F/gas 5.

Step two In a pan, heat the milk with the stock powder or cube. Dissolve the cornflour in a little cold water and stir into the sauce. Stir continuously as the sauce thickens, then reduce the heat and simmer for 2–3 minutes.

Step three Stir in the remaining ingredients, except the soy sauce and potatoes. Season well with salt and black pepper and pour into the base of an ovenproof dish.

Step four Cover with the sliced potatoes and drizzle with the soy sauce. Place near the top of the oven and bake for 35–40 minutes until golden brown.

Step five Garnish with whole chives, if using, and serve hot with a selection of fresh vegetables.

Serves 4

300ml (½ pint) skimmed milk

1 tablespoon vegetable stock powder or 1 vegetable stock cube

4 teaspoons cornflour

1 tablespoon Dijon mustard

50g (2oz) low-fat Cheddar, grated

115g (4oz) thinly sliced smoked ham, cut into strips

1 tablespoon chopped fresh chives

4 medium baking potatoes, thinly sliced

1 tablespoon light soy sauce

whole chives, to garnish (optional)

salt and freshly ground black pepper

per serving:

266 kcal/3.9g fat

Pot-roast Lamb with Celery and Peppers

A delicious lamb dish full of flavour. Choose a very lean piece of meat, as lamb is naturally high in fat. Other cuts of meat, such as silverside or topside of beef, are equally suited.

Serves 4

1kg (2¼ lb) leg of lamb, skin removed

2 garlic cloves, sliced

3–4 sprigs fresh rosemary

2 medium red onions, chopped

1 head celery, trimmed and sliced

2 red peppers, seeded and sliced

1.2 litres (2 pints) meat stock

2 tablespoons plain flour

2 tablespoons tomato purée

2 pieces lemon peel

salt and freshly ground black pepper

per serving:

353 kcal/13.5g fat

Step one Preheat the oven to 180°C/350°F/gas 4.

Step two Using a small, sharp knife, make incisions all over the lamb. Push slices of garlic and small sprigs of rosemary into the holes and season well with salt and black pepper.

Step three Preheat a non-stick frying pan until very hot. Add the lamb and quickly brown on all sides, then transfer the meat to an earthenware pot.

Step four Reduce the heat under the pan to medium and add the onions, celery and peppers. Cook until lightly coloured. Add 2–3 tablespoons of stock and sprinkle the flour over, cook briefly, then gradually mix in the remaining stock. If the pan is not sufficiently big enough to hold all the liquid, transfer the mixture to the earthenware pot and add the remaining stock, along with the tomato purée and lemon peel.

Step five Cover the pot and place in the preheated oven for 2–2½ hours until tender.

Step six Before serving, scoop off any fat from the top of the pot with a small ladle, then transfer the meat from the sauce onto a serving plate. Adjust the consistency of the sauce by reducing it in a pan over high heat. Serve with seasonal vegetables.

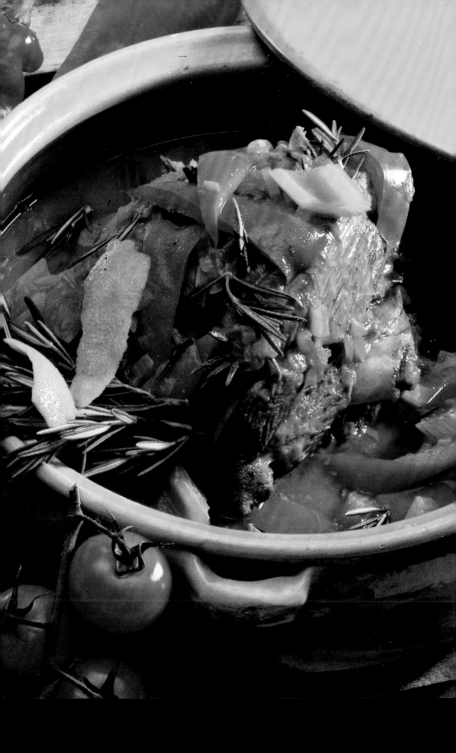

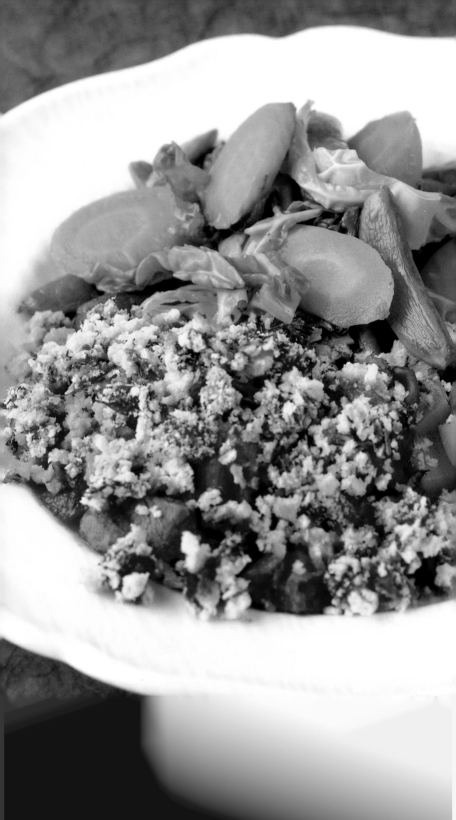

Lamb and Pepper Crumble

The crunchy topping in this recipe can be used on many different foods, such as fish or chicken. It's a good way of using up stale bread.

Step one Preheat the oven to 200°C/400°F/gas 6. Preheat a non-stick pan to a high heat.

Step two Trim away any traces of fat from the lamb, then season generously with salt and black pepper. Seal the meat on all sides in the hot pan.

Step three Add the onion, garlic and red pepper to the pan. Cook quickly over a high heat to soften. Add the tomato Passata, stock and herbs, stirring well. Cover and simmer for 20 minutes to allow the lamb to cook through.

Step four Meanwhile, place the breadcrumbs on a baking sheet and grill under a medium heat, turning them with a spatula, until well toasted. When toasted, place in a mixing bowl, add the chopped mint and mix in the cranberry sauce.

Step five Place the lamb in the base of an ovenproof dish and scatter the crumble on top. Bake in the oven for 20 minutes, and then serve with a selection of fresh vegetables.

Serves 6

1kg (2¼ lb) lean lamb, diced

1 medium red onion, finely chopped

2 garlic cloves, crushed

1 red pepper, seeded and finely chopped

600ml (1 pint) tomato Passata

2 teaspoons vegetable stock powder dissolved in 300ml (½ pint) water

1 tablespoon chopped fresh mixed herbs

115g (4oz) fresh breadcrumbs

2 tablespoons chopped fresh mint

2 tablespoons cranberry sauce

salt and freshly ground black pepper

per serving:
377 kcal/15g fat

107

Lamb Steaks Boulangères

This classic French dish is easy to prepare yet full of flavour. Serve it straight from the oven with plenty of seasonal vegetables. Choose potatoes suitable for baking. The waxy, firm type such as red Desirée is the best, as these will hold their shape and not break up during baking.

Serves 4

4 lean lamb steaks

2 medium onions, sliced

2 garlic cloves, crushed

1 tablespoon herbes de Provence

450g (1lb) potatoes, peeled and finely sliced

1.2 litres (2 pints) lamb stock

1 tablespoon cornflour

chopped fresh parsley, to garnish

salt and freshly ground black pepper

per serving:

296 kcal/8.1g fat

Step one Preheat the oven to 180°C/350°F/gas 4.

Step two Remove any fat from the lamb. Season each steak on both sides with salt and black pepper, then dry-fry in a non-stick frying pan over medium heat until sealed.

Step three Place the steaks in an ovenproof dish and cover with the onion and garlic. Sprinkle the herbs on top and cover with the sliced potatoes. Season well, then add the lamb stock. Cook in the oven for 1 hour.

Step four When the lamb is cooked, blend the cornflour with a little water and use to thicken the stock. Garnish with chopped parsley and serve immediately with a selection of fresh vegetables.

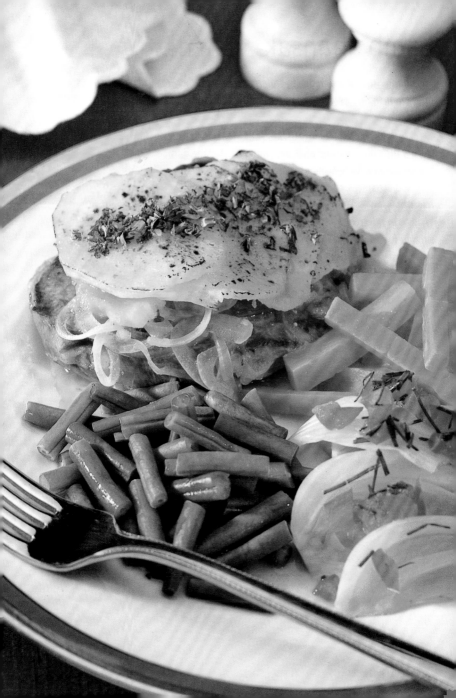

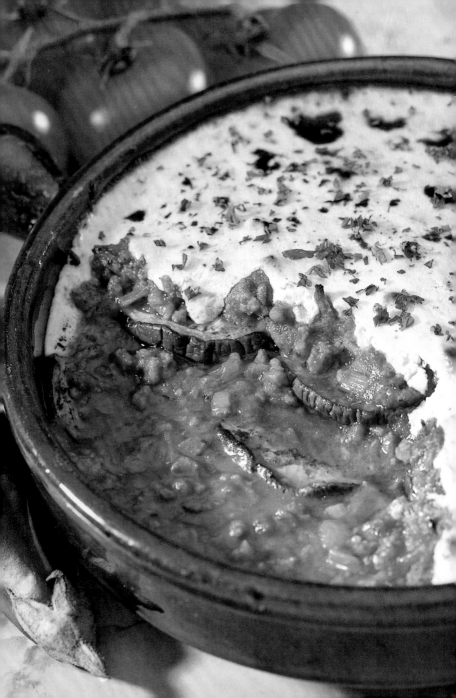

Moussaka

Traditional moussaka uses a heavy quota of oil. The sauce is usually started by frying the onion and meat. Then the aubergine slices are individually fried in oil, and this is all topped with a rich cheese sauce. This low-fat alternative is a treat for any palate. If you wish, you can prepare the aubergine in advance and store it sealed in a container in the refrigerator.

Step one Preheat the oven to 180°C/350°F/gas 4.

Step two Dry-fry the onion in a non-stick frying pan over medium heat until soft. Add the garlic and the lamb. Cook quickly until the meat is well sealed. Add the thyme, tomatoes and tomato purée. Simmer gently and season with salt and black pepper.

Step three Preheat a grill to medium heat. Cut the aubergine into thin slices, place on a non-stick baking sheet and season with plenty of salt and black pepper. Place under the preheated grill for 2–3 minutes on each side until golden.

Step four Place alternate layers of the lamb mixture and aubergine in an ovenproof dish. Combine the yoghurt with the beaten egg and the mustard, season well, and pour over the lamb.

Step five Bake for 30–35 minutes or until golden brown. Sprinkle over the chopped parsley and serve with a crisp green salad.

Serves 6

1 large onion, chopped

2 garlic cloves, crushed

450g (1lb) lean minced lamb

1 tablespoon chopped fresh thyme

1 x 400g (14oz) tin chopped tomatoes

1 tablespoon tomato purée

1 large aubergine

300ml (½ pint) low-fat natural yoghurt

1 egg, beaten

1 teaspoon English mustard powder

2 tablespoons chopped fresh parsley, to garnish

salt and freshly ground black pepper

per serving:
258 kcal/10g fat

Lamb's Liver with Orange Sauce

Liver and orange is a delightful combination. You could also try them together on kebabs with smoked bacon.

Serves 4

450g (1lb) lamb's liver

150ml (¼ pint) skimmed milk

1 onion, finely chopped

300ml (½ pint) freshly squeezed orange juice

1 teaspoon chopped fresh thyme

1 teaspoon arrowroot

salt and freshly ground black pepper

per serving:

177 kcal/6.4g fat

Step one Remove any membrane or veins from the liver. Place the liver in a bowl and cover with the milk. Leave to stand for 1–2 hours. This will remove any bitter flavours and keep the liver moist during cooking.

Step two Remove the liver from the milk and dry-fry over medium heat in a preheated non-stick frying pan, seasoning it well with salt and black pepper as you turn it over. Continue to dry-fry the liver until it is cooked but still slightly pink in the centre, then remove from the pan and keep warm.

Step three Add the onion to the pan and dry-fry over medium heat for 1 minute, scraping up any residue from the liver. Pour in the orange juice and add the thyme. Mix the arrowroot with a little cold water to form a paste. Pour this into the pan, stirring well, and simmer until the sauce thickens.

Step four Return the liver to the pan, turning it well to coat it with the sauce. Transfer to individual plates and serve immediately with potatoes and fresh seasonal vegetables of your choice.

If you like you can dress this dish up by garnishing it with a sprinkling of chopped parsley and a few slices of orange just before serving.

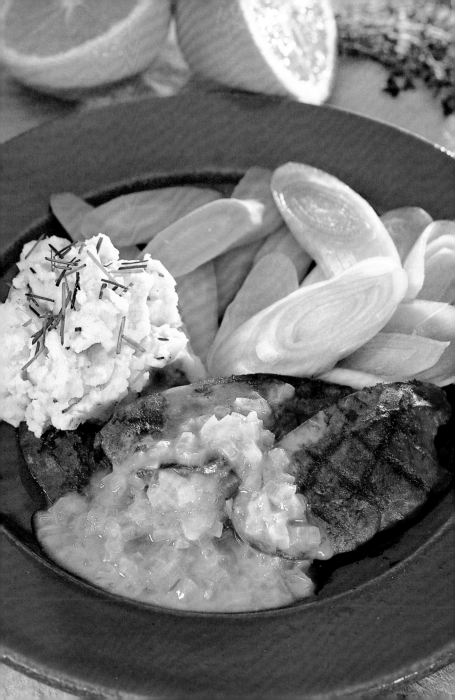

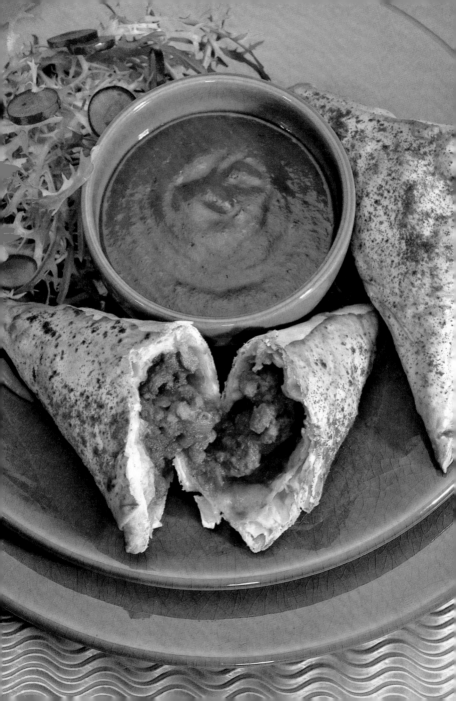

Lamb Samosas with Dipping Sauce

Traditionally, samosas are deep-fried, highly spiced pasties. In this recipe, the fat is reduced significantly by using filo pastry and then baking the pasties rather than frying them.

Step one Preheat a non-stick frying pan on medium heat, add the onion and garlic and dry-fry until soft. Add the minced lamb and continue cooking over a high heat to seal the meat.

Step two Sprinkle the curry powder over and 'cook out' for 1 minute, stirring well, then add the bouillon powder and Passata. Simmer gently for 15–20 minutes until the liquid has reduced to leave a thick paste. Allow to cool.

Step three Preheat the oven to 200°C/400°F/gas 6.

Step four Beat together the egg and the milk. Take a sheet of filo pastry and brush with the egg mixture. Fold a third of the long side into the centre and again on the other side to leave a long strip of pastry. Brush again with egg, then place a good tablespoon of the lamb mixture at one end of the pastry and fold over diagonally, enclosing the mixture in a triangle. Fold the pastry back over along the length of the pastry, retaining the triangle shape and tucking in any spare ends. Brush with egg, place on a baking tray and dust lightly with paprika. Repeat this process for the remaining seven parcels.

Step five Bake the samosas in the oven for 20–25 minutes until golden brown.

Step six Combine all the sauce ingredients in a small bowl and season with salt and black pepper. Serve the samosas on a bed of mixed salad leaves with the dipping sauce.

Makes 8

1 medium onion, finely diced

2 garlic cloves, crushed

225g (8oz) lean minced lamb

1 tablespoon curry powder

2 teaspoons vegetable bouillon powder

300ml (½ pint) tomato Passata

1 egg

3 tablespoons skimmed milk

8 sheets filo pastry

1 teaspoon paprika

for the dipping sauce

150ml (¼ pint) tomato Passata

1 tablespoon mango chutney

1 small red chilli, seeded and finely chopped

1 tablespoon chopped fresh coriander

salt and freshly ground black pepper

per samosa:
174 kcal/6.4g fat

Smoked Mackerel Salad Niçoise

The classic French Niçoise salad contains olives and anchovies in an oil-rich dressing. This low-fat alternative, while quite different, offers an interesting combination with good strong flavours.

Serves 4

115g (4oz) fine
green beans

450g (1lb) new
potatoes, cooked
and sliced

20 cherry tomatoes

350g (12oz) smoked
mackerel fillets

1 red onion,
finely chopped

20 small black
seedless grapes

for the dressing

2 tablespoons
lemon juice

1 tablespoon
balsamic vinegar

1 tablespoon
chopped fresh chives

1 teaspoon Dijon
mustard

salt and freshly ground
black pepper

per serving:

426 kcal/27g fat

Step one Cook the beans in salted boiling water until tender. Drain and refresh under cold running water.

Step two Slice the beans in half lengthways and place in a large bowl with the new potatoes. Slice the tomatoes in half and add to the bowl.

Step three Remove the skin from the mackerel and flake the mackerel into bite-sized pieces, checking for any bones. Add to the salad along with the red onion and grapes.

Step four Combine the dressing ingredients in a bowl. Pour over the salad and serve with crusty bread.

To make the salad even more substantial you can serve it on a bed of mixed salad leaves, either on a large platter or on individual plates.

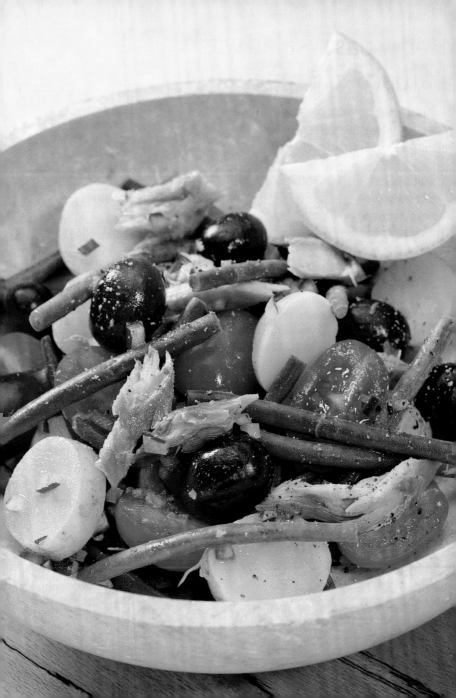

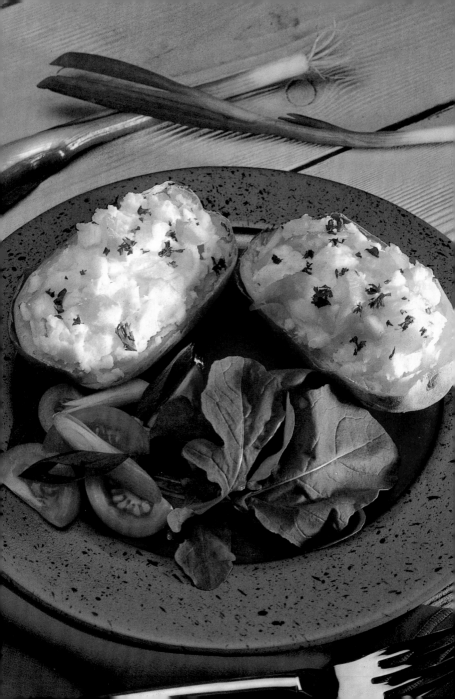

Smoked Haddock Boats

The subtle flavour of the baked potatoes and the fromage frais strike a perfect balance with the rich, smoky taste of the haddock. They keep the fat level and calorie count down too.

Step one Preheat the oven to 180°C/350°F/gas 4.

Step two Wash and prick the potatoes and bake in the oven for 1½–2 hours.

Step three When soft, cut each potato in half lengthways. Scoop the insides of each half into a bowl, leaving the skins intact. Add the fromage frais to the bowl and season with salt and black pepper. Stir in the smoked haddock and spoon the mixture back into the potato skins.

Step four Turn the oven up to 200°C/400°F/gas 6. Return the potatoes to the oven for a further 10–15 minutes. Just before serving, sprinkle with chopped parsley. Serve with a green salad and tomatoes.

Serves 4

4 large baking potatoes

2 tablespoons virtually fat-free fromage frais

100g (4oz) smoked haddock, cooked and flaked

chopped fresh parsley, to garnish

salt and freshly ground black pepper

per serving:

347 kcal/2g fat

Baked Sea Bass with Dill and Lemon Sauce

Sea bass is a firm, meaty fish with large, white flakes. It takes very little cooking and can easily dry out, so be cautious not to overcook it.

Serves 4

4 whole sea bass, gutted

300ml (½ pint) apple juice

juice of 1 lemon

2 teaspoons Dijon mustard

2 teaspoons finely chopped dill

½ teaspoon ground fennel seeds

1 teaspoon green peppercorns in brine

2 teaspoons arrowroot

2 tablespoons low-fat fromage frais

1 tablespoon chopped fresh mint

flat-leaf parsley, to garnish

salt and freshly ground black pepper

per serving:

210 kcal/4.8g fat

Step one Preheat the oven to 200°C/400°F/gas 6.

Step two Place the sea bass on a chopping board and score several times with a sharp knife. Season the fish well on both sides and place on a non-stick baking tray. Place in the centre of the oven for 10–15 minutes.

Step three Place the remaining ingredients, except the arrowroot, fromage frais, mint and parsley, in a small pan over medium heat, stirring continuously to combine. Bring the sauce to a low simmer. Mix the arrowroot with a little cold water and whisk into the sauce.

Step four Just before serving, remove the sauce from the heat and stir in the fromage frais and mint. Arrange the fish on individual plates and pour the sauce over each. Serve with fresh vegetables and garnish with flat-leaf parsley, if you like.

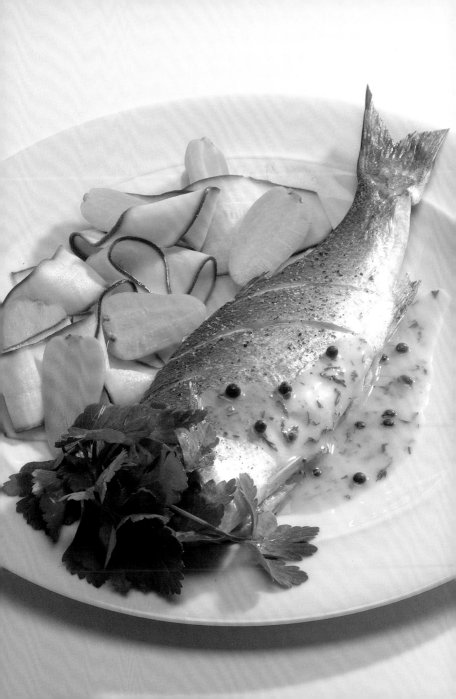

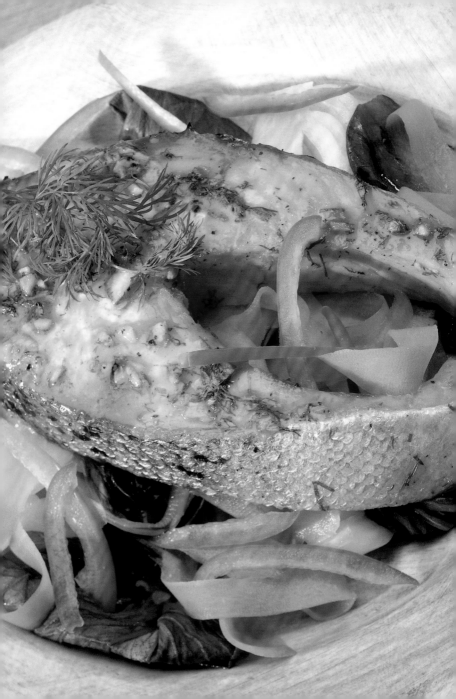

Baked Salmon with Sweet Ginger

Sweet and sour flavours enhance this quick and easy fish dish, which can also be cooked under a hot grill for 6–8 minutes, depending on the thickness of the fish. Check that it is cooked by carefully pulling the flesh apart, using two knives. The flesh inside should be light pink in colour and not wet in appearance. When cooked, the flesh will flake away from the skin easily.

Step one Preheat the oven to 200°C/400°F/gas 6.

Step two First make the glaze by combining the lemon juice, sugar, ginger, dill and soy sauce in a bowl. Season it with salt and black pepper.

Step three Place a salmon steak in the bowl and toss in the glaze. Repeat with the remaining 3 steaks. Transfer the salmon to an ovenproof dish and pour the glaze over.

Step four Bake for 8–10 minutes until just cooked. Serve with salad or seasonal vegetables.

Serves 4

4 salmon steaks

for the glaze

2 tablespoons lemon juice

4 teaspoons light muscovado sugar

1 teaspoon finely chopped fresh ginger

4 teaspoons chopped fresh dill

4 teaspoons light soy sauce

salt and freshly ground black pepper

per serving:

173 kcal/10g fat

Trout and Spinach Paupiettes with Dill and Cucumber Sauce

These are quick and easy to prepare. Ask a fishmonger to skin the fillets and be sure to remove any bones with a clean pair of tweezers.

Serves 4

225g (8oz) packet baby spinach

75g (3oz) 0 per cent fat Greek-style yoghurt

freshly grated nutmeg

2 x 225g (8oz) skinned, filleted trout, cut in half lengthways

2 tablespoons fresh lemon juice

2 slices lemon

2 sprigs fresh dill

salt and freshly ground black pepper

for the sauce

150ml (¼ pint) well-flavoured fish or vegetable stock

2 tablespoons dry white wine (optional)

1 x 100g (4oz) piece cucumber, halved and thinly sliced

2 level teaspoons cornflour

2 tablespoons chopped fresh dill

2 extra lemon slices, to garnish (optional)

per serving:

365 kcal/13.2g fat

Step one Preheat the oven to 220°C/425°F/gas 7. Blanch the spinach for 45–60 seconds. Place in a colander and rinse quickly with cold water. Drain, then squeeze to dry. Chop it and place it in a bowl. Add 3 tablespoons of the yoghurt, season to taste with salt, black pepper and nutmeg, and mix well.

Step two Place the fillets, skinned-side up, on a board. Season and spread some spinach over each one. Roll up each fillet from the head end to the tail and secure with a cocktail stick.

Step three Place the paupiettes in a small ovenproof dish and sprinkle with the lemon juice. Add the lemon slices and dill sprigs, then cover the dish tightly with foil. Place in the centre of the oven. Bake for 8–10 minutes, or until the trout turn opaque and the flesh flakes easily, but do not let them dry out.

Step four Meanwhile, make the sauce. Pour the stock into a small pan, add the white wine, if using, and the cucumber. Bring to the boil, then reduce the heat, partially cover the pan with a lid and gently simmer for 2–3 minutes until the cucumber is slightly soft.

Step five Blend the cornflour with 2 teaspoons of water and stir it into the cucumber sauce. Add the chopped dill and bring to the boil, stirring continuously, until the sauce thickens slightly. Reduce the heat and simmer for 1–2 minutes. Stir in the remaining yogurt, season, and cook for a further minute.

Step six Remove the cocktail sticks from the paupiettes, then carefully remove the paupiettes from the ovenproof dish and arrange on warmed plates. Pour over the cucumber and dill sauce, garnish with lemon slices (if using) and serve.

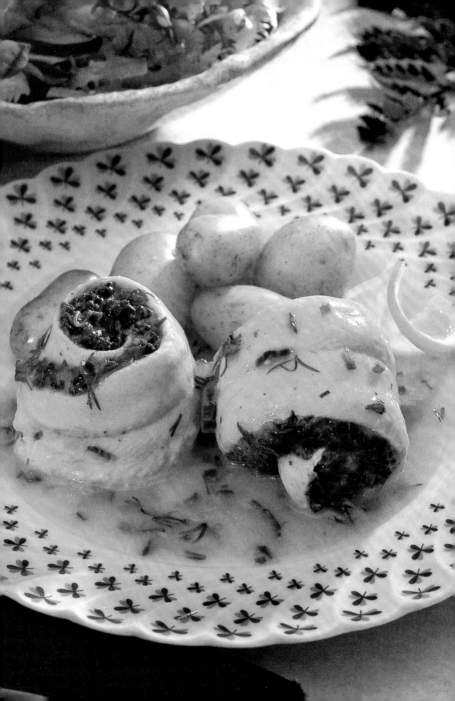

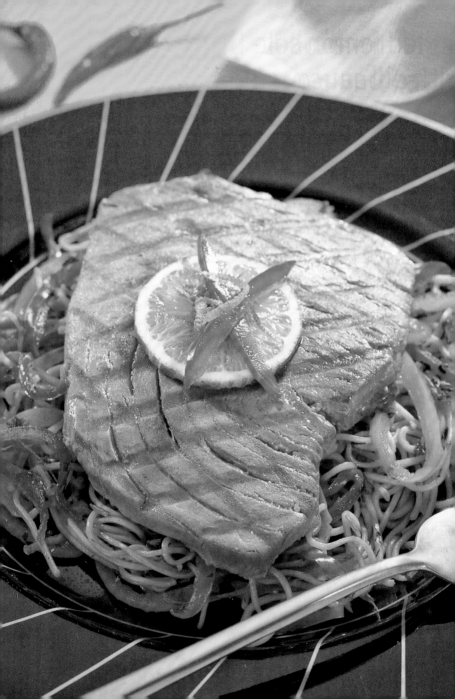

Pan-fried Tuna with Pepper Noodles

Fresh tuna tastes completely different from tinned tuna. Its lean, meaty flesh holds together well, making it ideal to pan-fry or even barbecue. It benefits from being served slightly underdone, with a moist centre.

Step one Trim the tuna steaks with a sharp knife, removing any unsightly dark flesh. Season well with salt and black pepper.

Step two Prepare the noodles by placing them in boiling salted water for 2–3 minutes. Then drain and refresh them under cold running water.

Step three Heat a griddle pan or non-stick frying pan on medium heat, add the vegetable oil and then wipe out the pan with a piece of kitchen paper, taking care not to burn your fingers (use an oven glove if necessary).

Step four Place the tuna, best-side down, in the hot pan. As the tuna cooks it will change colour. Rather like a thermometer, the colour band will change and move up the fish. When it reaches halfway up the steaks, turn them over and cook for a minute or so more. Remove from the pan and place in a warm oven to keep hot.

Step five Add the garlic and peppers to the pan and quickly sauté over medium heat until they start to soften. Add the noodles, lime zest and juice and soy sauce. Cook for 1–2 minutes, turning regularly.

Step six Place the noodles on warmed serving plates and set the tuna on top. Garnish each one with a slice of lime and some finely sliced red pepper.

Serves 4

4 fresh tuna steaks

225g (8oz) fine egg noodles

1 teaspoon vegetable oil

1 garlic clove, crushed

1 red pepper, seeded and finely sliced

1 yellow pepper, seeded and finely sliced

zest and juice of 1 lime

1 tablespoon light soy sauce

4 lime slices and finely sliced red pepper, to garnish

salt and freshly ground black pepper

per serving:

356 kcal/8.6g fat

Salmon and Broccoli Lasagne

This recipe can be made in advance and cooked as required. It is suitable for home freezing.

Serves 4

225g (8oz) broccoli, trimmed

4 x 175g (6oz) salmon fillets

600ml (1 pint) skimmed milk

2 teaspoons Dijon mustard

2 teaspoons vegetable bouillon stock powder

2 tablespoons cornflour

115g (4oz) chestnut mushrooms, sliced

50g (2oz) low-fat Cheddar, grated

1 tablespoon chopped fresh dill

1 tablespoon chopped fresh parsley

225g (8oz) 'no cook' lasagne

flat-leaf parsley sprigs and lemon slices, to garnish

salt and freshly ground black pepper

Step one Preheat the oven to 190°C/375°F/gas 5. Cook the broccoli in boiling salted water, drain and set aside.

Step two Place the salmon in a pan with the milk and cook gently over a low heat for 5–6 minutes. Let cool, then lift out the fish onto a plate and flake, removing all skin and bones.

Step three Reheat the milk over medium-low heat, adding the mustard and stock powder to the pan. Slake the cornflour with a little cold water and add to the milk, stirring well to stop lumps forming.

Step four Add the mushrooms and cheese and mix well. Gently simmer until the sauce is of a coating consistency. Adjust if necessary with a little extra milk or diluted cornflour. Stir in the herbs.

Step five Place a thin layer of sauce in the base of an ovenproof dish. Cover with sheets of lasagne without overlapping them. Add a layer of flaked fish and broccoli then continue layering, ending with the sauce.

Step six Bake for 30–35 minutes until bubbling hot. Serve the lasagne garnished with slices of lemon and a few sprigs of flat-leaf parsley.

per serving:
658 kcal/23g fat

For a video masterclass on filleting salmon, go to
www.mykitchentable.co.uk/videos/filleting

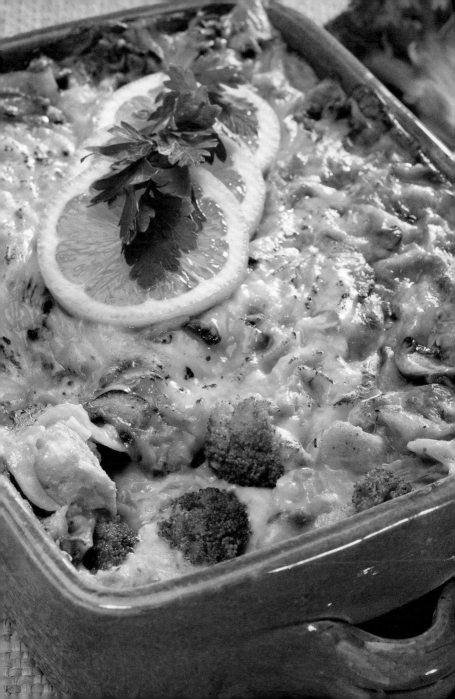

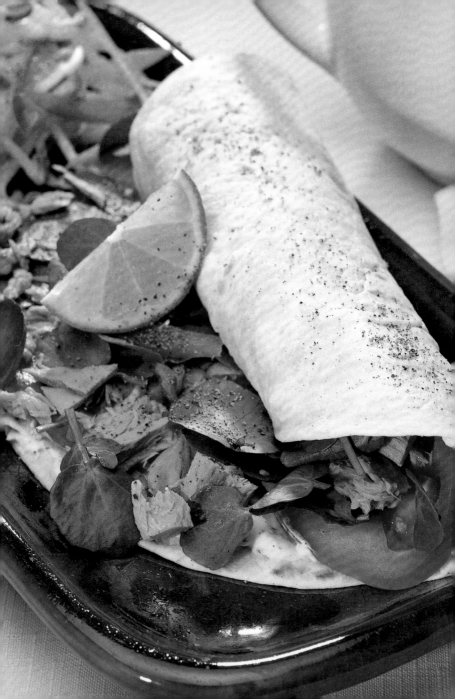

Lime Tuna Roll-ups

Creamy, low-fat cheese flavoured with garlic makes the ideal base for these rolls. You can vary the fillings by using cooked ham or roasted vegetables and even slice the roll-ups into finger food for parties.

Step one In a small bowl, combine the quark, garlic, chives and lime juice, season well with salt and black pepper, and mix together.

Step two Place the pitta breads on a chopping board and spread with the quark mixture. Cover with the tomato slices, tuna and watercress. Roll up tightly, and secure with wooden cocktail sticks if necessary.

Step three Chill until ready to serve.

Serves 4

225g (8oz) quark
low-fat soft cheese

1 smoked garlic
clove, crushed

2 tablespoons snipped
fresh chives

juice of 1 lime

4 large flat
pitta breads

2 ripe tomatoes, sliced

1 x 200g (7oz) tin tuna
steak in brine, drained

1 bunch watercress,
washed

salt and freshly ground
black pepper

per serving:

194 kcal/0.9g fat

Seafood Pie

The fish starts off uncooked, so it is essential that the pie is cooked in a hot oven to get the heat through to the centre of the pie. If the pie starts to brown too quickly, cover the top with foil and place lower in the oven to finish cooking. To dress the dish up for special occasions or a dinner party you can garnish it with cooked prawns in the shell and lemon slices.

Serves 6

675g (1½ lb) potatoes, peeled

2 tablespoons virtually fat-free fromage frais

225g (8oz) smoked haddock

225g (8oz) peeled prawns

115g (4oz) smoked or cooked mussels (optional)

225g (8oz) crab meat

2 baby leeks, chopped

150ml (¼ pint) fish stock

1 tablespoon plain flour

½ wine glass white wine or sherry

2–3 teaspoons mild Dijon mustard

600ml (1 pint) skimmed milk

1 tablespoon snipped fresh chives

chopped fresh parsley, to garnish

salt and freshly ground black pepper

per serving:
283 kcal/3.5g fat

Step one Preheat the oven to 220°C/425°F/gas 7.

Step two Boil the potatoes in a pan of salted water until well cooked. Drain and mash well until smooth. Add the fromage frais and season well.

Step three Remove the skin and bones from the smoked haddock and place in the base of an ovenproof dish. Add the prawns and the mussels, if using. Check the crab meat for pieces of shell or tendons and place on top.

Step four Place the leeks and the fish stock in a medium-sized pan and cook for 1–2 minutes. Sprinkle the flour over and mix well. 'Cook out' for 1 minute over a low heat, then add the white wine and mustard, beating well. Gradually add the skimmed milk, stirring continuously to prevent any lumps forming. Bring to the boil, allowing the sauce to thicken.

Step five Pour the sauce over the fish and allow to cool, stirring in the chives. Cover with the mashed potatoes, using either a fork or a piping bag with a large star nozzle.

Step six Bake in the oven for 30–40 minutes until golden. Garnish with chopped parsley and serve.

The sauce may boil over the sides of the dish while it is cooking, so line the base of the oven with foil for easy cleaning later.

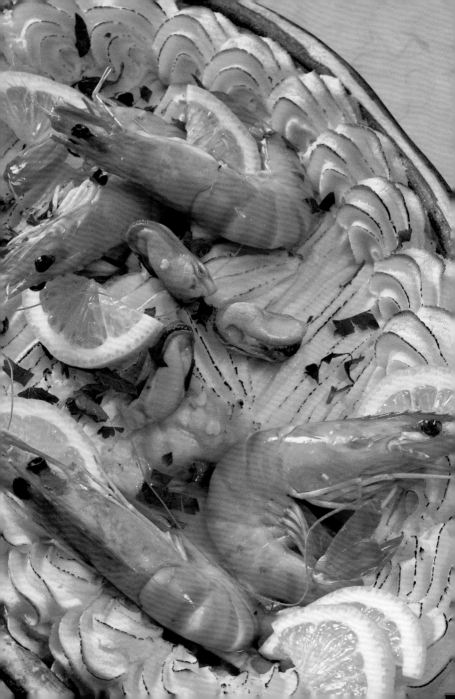

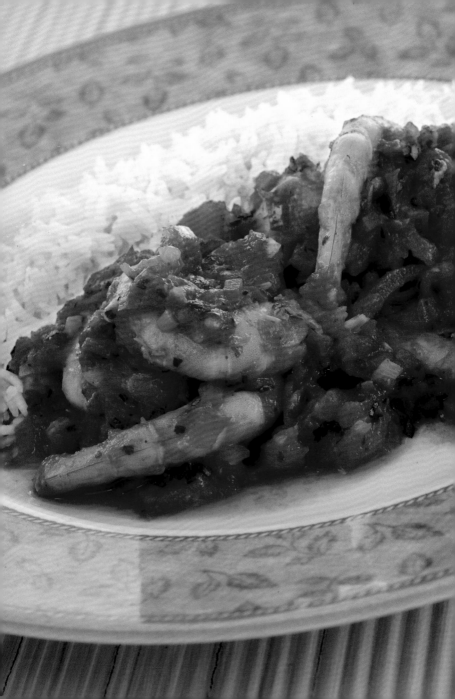

Arrabbiata prawns

These hot and spicy prawns also make a great baked potato topping if you fancy a change from rice.

Step one Rinse the prawns well under cold, running water.

Step two Preheat a non-stick frying pan. Add the onion and dry-fry over medium heat for 2–3 minutes until soft. Add the garlic and red pepper and cook for 2–3 minutes more.

Step three Add the prawns and cook for 5–6 minutes. Add the tomatoes and chilli, bringing the sauce to a gentle simmer. The prawns should be firm and cooked through.

Step four Season to taste with salt and black pepper. Add the basil leaves and serve with boiled rice.

Serves 4

225g (8oz) uncooked peeled prawns

1 red onion, finely chopped

2 garlic cloves, crushed

1 red pepper, seeded and finely diced

1 x 400g (14oz) tin chopped tomatoes

1 red chilli, seeded and finely chopped

8–10 basil leaves

salt and freshly ground black pepper

per serving:

87 kcal/0.7g fat

Paella

Traditionally, paella is cooked in a large, shallow pan with handles on both sides. This recipe will fill a 30–35cm (12–14in) pan. If you are unable to find prepared squid, see page 144 to read how to do it yourself.

Serves 6

275g (10oz) prepared squid tails or 450g (1lb) monkfish or 275g (10oz) firm fish fillets

450g (1lb) mussels

6–8 prawns, in shells

4 boneless, skinless chicken breasts

1 onion, chopped

1 leek, finely sliced

4 garlic cloves, crushed

900ml (1½ pints) fish or chicken stock

350g (12oz) arborio rice, rinsed in water

1 red pepper, seeded and diced

4 medium tomatoes, diced

100g (4oz) frozen peas

2 good pinches saffron

chopped fresh parsley and 2 lemons, cut into wedges, to garnish

salt and freshly ground black pepper

per serving:

417 kcal/8.8g fat

Step one Preheat the oven to 160°C/325°F/gas 3. Cut the prepared squid into rings and any tentacles in half. Remove the membrane from the outside of the monkfish (if using). Cut through the fish from the thin side and away from the bone, then cut the flesh into medallions about 1cm (½in) thick.

Step two Wash the mussels in several changes of water. Throw away any that are damaged or remain open when immersed in cold water. Scrub them well, scrape off any barnacles, pull off the 'beards' and wash them well again. You can remove the heads from the prawns, though the tradition is to keep them on.

Step three Dry-fry the chicken on medium heat in a preheated pan until coloured. Remove from the pan. Add the onion, leek, garlic and stock to the pan and gently simmer for 5–6 minutes.

Step four Stir the rice into the stock. Add the red pepper, tomatoes, peas and the saffron. Mix well and season to taste with salt and black pepper. Stir in the squid and fish and arrange the chicken, mussels and prawns evenly on top.

Step five Cover tightly and place in the preheated oven for 30–35 minutes until the rice and chicken are tender and all the liquid has been absorbed. It is important NOT to stir the rice while it is in the oven or it will cook unevenly. To test if it is cooked, take a grain or two carefully from the centre of the pan.

Step six When it is done, remove the pan from the oven. Cover it with damp greaseproof paper and leave for 4–5 minutes.

Step seven Just before serving, sprinkle the chopped parsley over the dish and garnish with the lemon wedges.

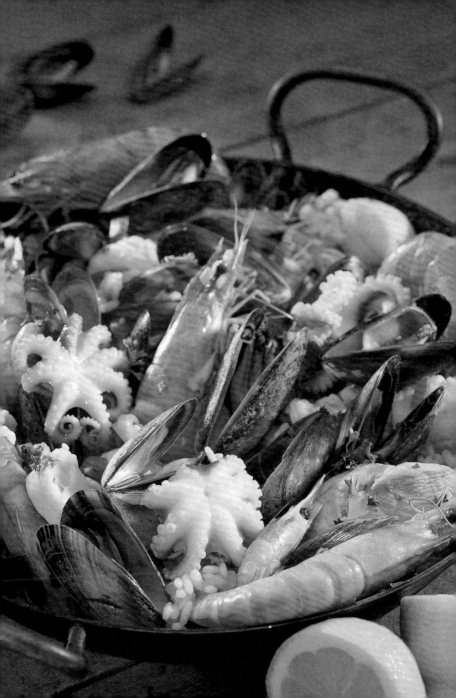

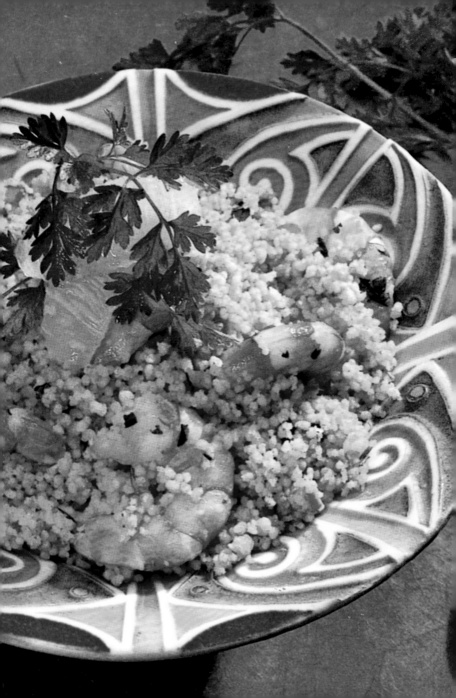

Chilli Prawn Couscous

Prawns take very little cooking. They are perfect when lightly steamed, as in this recipe, since they pick up the flavours from the spiced couscous. Alternatively, you could use white crab meat.

Step one In a medium pan, bring the vegetable stock to the boil. Add the spices, garlic, chilli and tomatoes.

Step two Gradually add the couscous, stirring well. Stir the prawns into the mixture. Cover with a tight-fitting lid and remove from the heat for 1 minute.

Step three Fluff up the couscous with 2 forks. Add the coriander, garnish with the lemon wedges and sprigs of flat-leaf parsley and serve immediately.

Serves 4

450ml (¾ pint) vegetable stock

¼ teaspoon fennel seeds

¼ teaspoon ground cumin

¼ teaspoon ground coriander

2 garlic cloves, crushed

1 small red chilli, seeded and finely chopped

1 x 225g (8oz) tin chopped tomatoes

450g (1lb) couscous

225g (8oz) uncooked peeled prawns

1 tablespoon chopped fresh coriander

lemon wedges and sprigs of flat-leaf parsley, to garnish

per serving:
313 kcal/1.8g fat

Steamed Sesame Prawn Balls with Lime Dip

This unusual dish is ideal as a light lunch or as a starter. It can be made in advance and kept in the refrigerator until ready to cook and serve. For a less spicy taste, you can substitute ground coriander or a pinch of nutmeg for the garam masala.

Serves 6

450g (1lb) uncooked prawns, shelled and deveined

4 spring onions, finely chopped

½ teaspoon garam masala

1 teaspoon shrimp paste

115g (4oz) ground rice

2 tablespoons finely chopped fresh coriander

2 tablespoons sesame seeds

sliced spring onions, to garnish

for the lime dip

1 tablespoon fish or vegetable stock

small pinch of saffron

150ml (¼ pint) virtually fat-free fromage frais

finely grated zest and juice of 2 limes

salt and freshly ground black pepper

Step one Place the prawns, spring onions, garam masala and shrimp paste in a food processor and mix until smooth. Scrape the mixture into a bowl and add the ground rice and coriander. Mix well until combined and season with salt and black pepper.

Step two Divide the mixture into small balls, then, using wet hands, roll until smooth and dip in the sesame seeds. Place on a plate, cover with clingfilm and chill until ready to cook.

Step three To make the lime dip, heat the stock with the saffron and allow the saffron to infuse for 2–3 minutes. Place the remaining dip ingredients into a serving bowl. Add the warm saffron-infused stock and mix to combine. Season to taste with salt and black pepper, then cover and chill until ready to serve.

Step four Place the prawn balls in a steamer over boiling water and cook, covered, for 3–4 minutes. Serve immediately, garnished with sliced spring onions and accompanied by the lime dip.

per serving:
162 kcal/4.8g fat

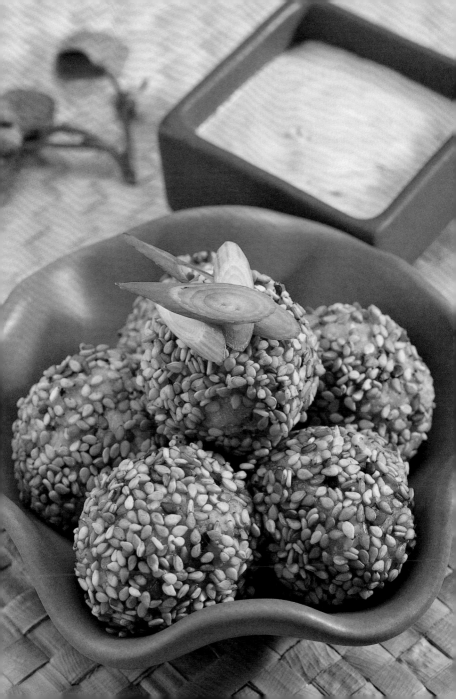

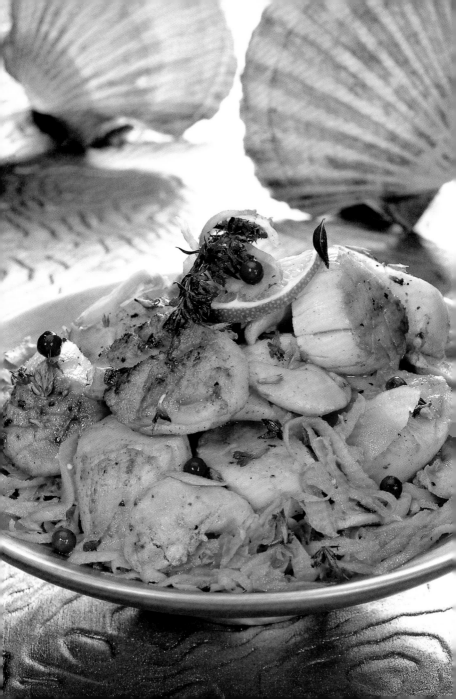

Seared Scallops with Carrot and Pink Ginger Pickle

Scallops make an ideal starter, as they are quite fleshy in appearance yet light and delicate in both volume and flavour. Make the carrot salad in advance and chill until ready to serve.

Step one Prepare the scallops by cleaning well under a cold running tap to remove any sand or grit. Pull away the small membrane attached to the side, being careful to keep the orange coral intact. Pat dry with kitchen towel and season well with salt and black pepper.

Step two Using the coarse side of a grater, grate the carrot into a bowl and add the crushed coriander seeds, peppercorns, ginger and vinegar. Season well, mixing the ingredients together. Mix in the fresh coriander and allow to stand for a minimum of 30 minutes.

Step three Preheat a non-stick griddle pan or frying pan on medium heat. Add a little vegetable oil, then wipe out, using a good pad of kitchen paper. Add the scallops to the pan and cook quickly for 1 minute on each side.

Step four Arrange the carrot salad on a serving plate. Squeeze the lime over the scallops and remove from the heat. Place on top of the carrot salad, pouring the pan juices over. Serve immediately, with crusty bread.

Serves 4

12–16 large
fresh scallops

225g (8oz) young
carrots, peeled

½ teaspoon coriander
seeds, crushed

¼ teaspoon pink
peppercorns

2 teaspoons Chinese
pink ginger, finely
sliced

1 tablespoon white
wine or fruit vinegar

1 tablespoon chopped
fresh coriander

a little vegetable oil

1 lime, sliced in half

salt and freshly ground
black pepper

per serving:
102 kcal/1.3g fat

Marinated Griddled Squid

Squid is very messy and can be time-consuming to prepare, so ask your fishmonger to clean them, or buy them ready prepared. Squid rings are available, but they do not have the full flavour that fresh squid has.

Serves 4

4 baby squid

2 teaspoons oil
(to line pan)

for the marinade

4 tablespoons
light soy sauce

zest and juice
of 2 limes

1 small red chilli,
seeded and finely
chopped

1 x 2.5cm (1in)
piece fresh ginger,
finely chopped

salt and freshly ground
black pepper

per serving:

102 kcal/2g fat

Step one If the squid is not already prepared, pull the head and tentacles away from the tail section. Cut the tentacles just above the eyes and discard the rest of the head. Cut away the round cartilage from the base of the tentacles and discard. Remove any reddish-brown membrane and rinse the squid well under cold water. Rinse the tail section under cold water, removing the inner, semi-transparent 'pen' and any reddish membrane from the outside. Place the squid on a chopping board and slice open from top to bottom, then rinse again to remove any inner membrane.

Step two Using a sharp knife, score both sides of the squid flesh in a diagonal pattern and place in a shallow dish. Combine all the marinade ingredients in a small bowl and pour over the squid. Leave to marinate for 30 minutes.

Step three Preheat a non-stick griddle pan or frying pan, lightly greasing with a little oil and then removing the excess with kitchen paper, taking care not to burn your fingers. When the pan is very hot, carefully add the squid, cooking it quickly for 1–2 minutes each side. Take care not to overcook it, as the texture will become tough and rubbery. When it is ready, serve the squid hot with salad leaves, rice or noodles.

For more recipes from My Kitchen Table, sign up for our newsletter at www.mykitchentable.co.uk/newsletter

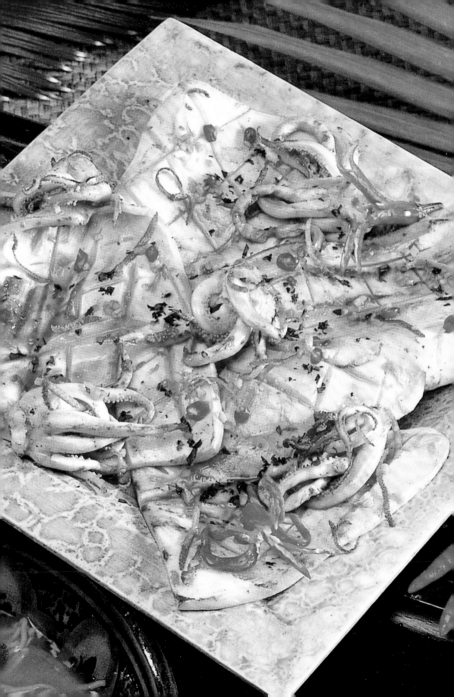

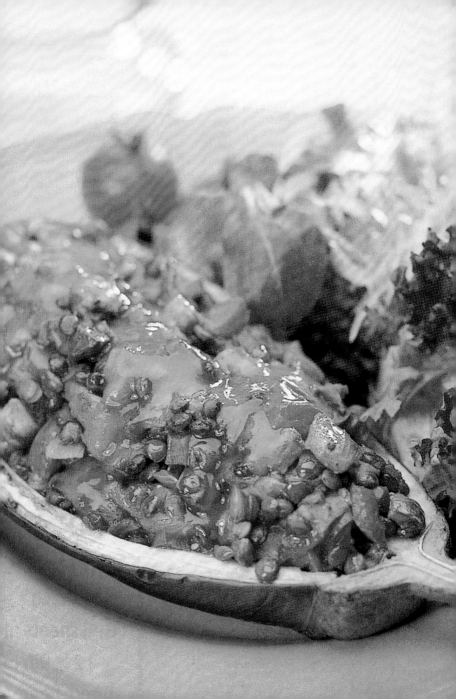

Stuffed Aubergine

This recipe can be used as a main course and served with unlimited salad or vegetables. Choose smooth-skinned, fresh aubergines, since wrinkled or bruised ones may be old and leathery.

Step one Cut the aubergines in half lengthways. Scoop out the flesh and sprinkle the insides and the flesh with salt. Leave to stand for 20 minutes. Rinse well and chop the flesh.

Step two Meanwhile, cook the lentils in boiling water for 25–30 minutes until tender. Drain.

Step three Preheat the oven to 180°C/350°F/gas 4.

Step four Place the oil in a pan over medium heat. Add the onion and sauté for 5 minutes until it begins to soften. Add the chopped aubergine, pepper and mushrooms and sauté for 5 minutes. Stir in the mustard and herbs and season well with salt and black pepper.

Step five Drain the tomatoes, reserving the juice. Chop the tomato flesh and add to the pan with the cooked lentils. Spoon into the aubergine shells. Bake for 45 minutes until the aubergines are tender.

Step six Just before the end of cooking time, stir a little tomato juice into the cornflour to form a smooth paste. Add the stock and juice. Heat gently, stirring continuously, until thickened. Season to taste and pour the sauce over the aubergines. Serve with a mixed green salad.

Serves 4

2 large aubergines

100g (4oz) [dry weight] Puy lentils, soaked

1 teaspoon olive oil

1 onion, finely chopped

1 red pepper, seeded and finely chopped

100g (4oz) mushrooms, chopped

1 teaspoon wholegrain mustard

1 teaspoon chopped mixed herbs

1 x 400g (14oz) tin tomatoes

2 teaspoons cornflour

150ml (¼ pint) vegetable stock

salt and freshly ground black pepper

per serving:

162 kcal/1.8g fat

Grilled Polenta with Wild Mushrooms

Polenta is coarsely ground maize. Bramata is the best quality and is rather like a coarse flour. Like pasta, it is a good base for incorporating many flavours. Since it is fat-free, it makes an ideal alternative to rice or potatoes and is available ready-made or part-cooked as an instant polenta. However, to get the authentic flavour, it is best made from scratch, using bramata polenta flour. A large batch can be frozen in pieces and then cooked from frozen as required.

Serves 4

225g (8oz) bramata polenta flour

1.2 litres (2 pints) vegetable stock

1 tablespoon chopped fresh sage

2 garlic cloves, crushed

1 medium shallot, finely diced

450g (1lb) fresh mixed wild mushrooms (e.g. oyster, shiitake, ceps)

juice of 1 lemon

1 tablespoon light soy sauce

1 tablespoon chopped fresh parsley, plus extra to garnish

salt and freshly ground black pepper

per serving:

231 kcal/2.4g fat

Step one Weigh the polenta flour into a large jug so that it can be poured easily. Place the stock in a large pan. Add the sage and half the garlic and bring to the boil. Slowly add the polenta in a continuous stream, stirring with a whisk to prevent lumps forming. Beat the mixture well, using a wooden spoon, until combined.

Step two Reduce the heat and simmer for 40–45 minutes until the polenta starts to leave the sides of the pan. Pour into a shallow dish or baking tin and allow to cool and set.

Step three In a non-stick frying pan, dry-fry the shallot over medium heat with the remaining garlic until soft. Add the mushrooms and cook for 2–3 minutes, seasoning well with salt and plenty of black pepper. Add the lemon juice, soy sauce and most of the parsley and simmer for 1–2 minutes.

Step four Cut the set polenta into squares and place face-down onto a baking sheet. Grill under a high heat for 1–2 minutes until golden brown. Spoon the mushroom mixture onto the polenta and sprinkle with the remainder of the chopped parsley.

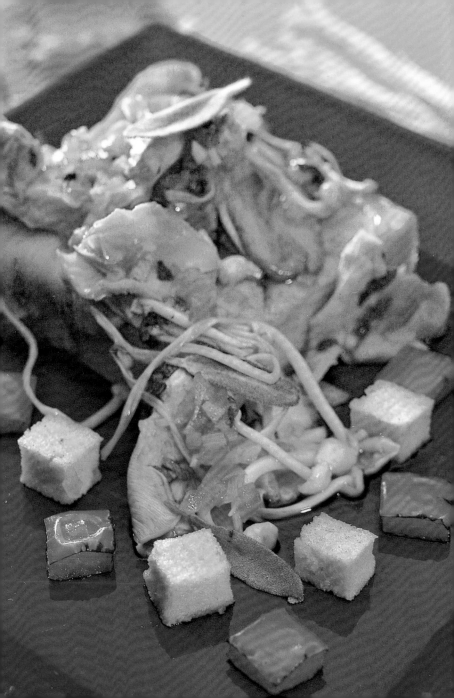

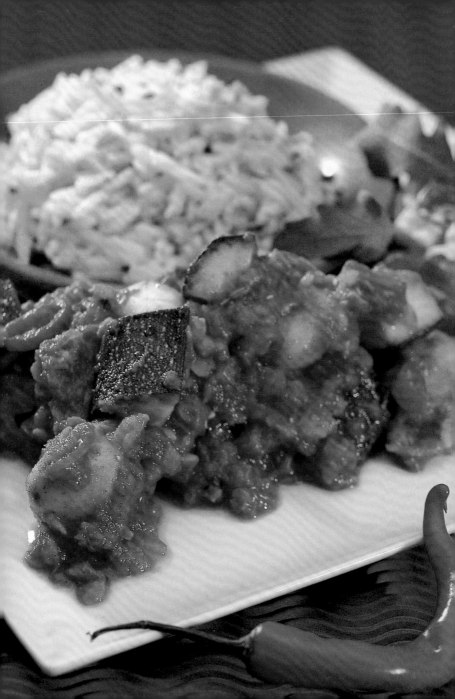

Leek and Courgette Dhansak

A dhansak is an Indian curry traditionally made with meat and thickened with lentils. The dish is usually started by frying the onion in ghee or butter. Here, we replace the meat and the fat with a selection of fresh vegetables. When combined with spices, it gives a really tasty vegetarian dish. You could use any seasonal vegetable (cauliflower works really well).

Step one Prepare the potatoes, leeks and courgettes by chopping into bite-sized pieces.

Step two Dry-fry the onions and garlic in a non-stick pan over medium heat until soft. Add the potatoes, leeks, courgettes and red pepper and cook for 2–3 minutes.

Step three Add the spices and the chillies, stirring well to coat the vegetables, and cook for a further minute in order to 'cook out' the spices.

Step four Add the lentils and stir the stock and tomato purée into the mixture. Season well with salt and black pepper. Cover and simmer for 35–40 minutes.

Step five Serve with boiled rice spiced with a little lemon zest, and a simple cucumber yoghurt salad.

Serves 4

450g (1lb) small waxy potatoes

225g (8oz) young leeks, washed

225g (8oz) small courgettes

2 medium onions, chopped

2 garlic cloves, crushed

1 red pepper, seeded and diced

1 tablespoon ground coriander

1 tablespoon ground cinnamon

1 tablespoon ground cumin

1 tablespoon fennel seeds

2 fresh green chillies, seeded and chopped

100g (4oz) red lentils

600ml (1 pint) vegetable stock

3 tablespoons tomato purée

salt and freshly ground black pepper

per serving:
302 kcal/3g fat

The Easiest Vegetable Pie Ever

As the name suggests, this vegetable pie is foolproof. It can be made in individual pie dishes or served as a hearty centrepiece.

Serves 4

1 x 750g (1¾lb) bag frozen mixed vegetables

175g (6oz) frozen cauliflower

100g (4oz) frozen peas

3 tablespoons cornflour

300ml (½ pint) skimmed milk

½ vegetable stock cube

65g (2½oz) half-fat vegetarian Cheddar, grated

4–5 sheets filo pastry

2 teaspoons sunflower oil

salt and freshly ground black pepper

per serving:

260 kcal/5.7g fat

Step one Preheat the oven to 200°C/400°F/gas 6.

Step two Bring a large pan of water to the boil, add all the frozen vegetables and return to the boil. Cook for 3–4 minutes. Drain, reserving 300ml (½ pint) of the cooking liquid. Place the vegetables in an ovenproof pie dish.

Step three Mix the cornflour with a little of the milk to form a paste, then stir in the remaining milk and the reserved vegetable water. Crumble the stock cube into the liquid. Cook gently in a pan, stirring continuously, until the sauce has thickened. Alternatively, cook in a microwave on High for 3–4 minutes, whisking once or twice during the cooking time.

Step four Stir the cheese into the sauce and season well, then pour over the vegetables.

Step five Brush each sheet of filo with a little oil, scrunch up slightly and place on top of the vegetables. Repeat until all the vegetables are covered. Bake for 20 minutes or until the pastry is golden. Serve with new potatoes and salad.

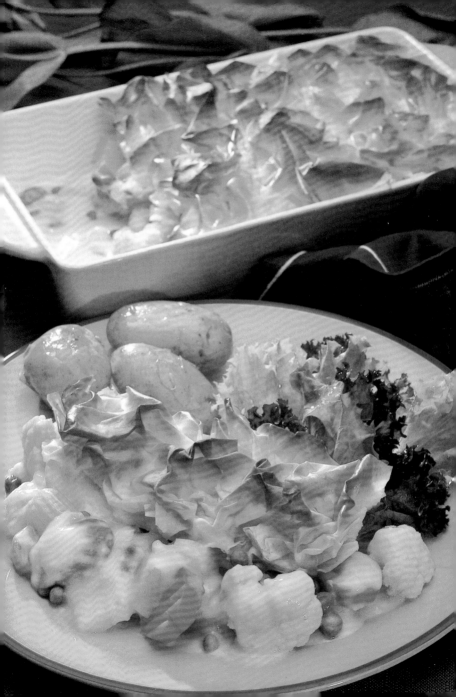

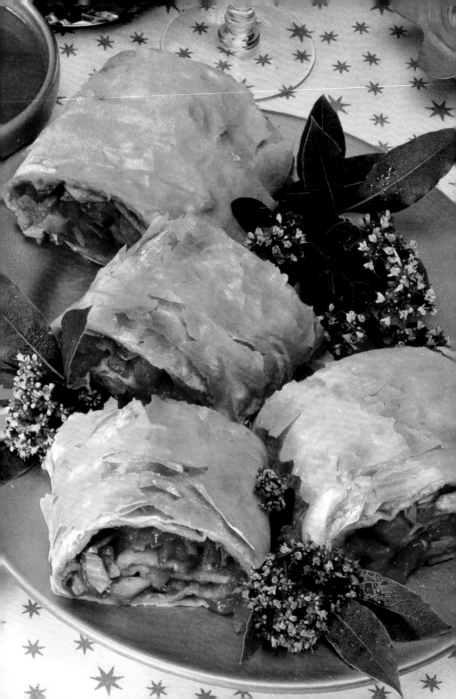

Roasted Pepper and Leek Strudel

A great vegetarian dish packed full of flavour. It can be frozen cooked or uncooked. Vary the filling by using different combinations of cooked or roasted vegetables and serve with a simple, spicy tomato sauce.

Step one Preheat the oven to 200°C/400°F/gas 6.

Step two Cut the peppers in half, remove the seeds, and place face down in a non-stick baking tin. Roast in the top of the oven for 20–30 minutes until soft. Remove from the oven and place inside a plastic food bag. Seal the bag and leave to cool.

Step three Preheat a non-stick frying pan and dry-fry the leeks over medium heat with the thyme and garlic until soft. Remove from the heat and stir in the basil, stock powder and Passata.

Step four Peel the cooled peppers, roughly chop and add to the leeks.

Step five Separate the filo pastry sheets. Place one onto a non-stick baking sheet and brush with the beaten egg. Continue adding the remaining sheets, brushing each layer with egg.

Step six Spread the leek and pepper filling over the pastry, leaving a 2.5cm (1in) border around the edge. Fold in the two short sides and roll up like a Swiss roll. Brush the top with egg and bake for 8–10 minutes, until crisp and golden.

Step seven Now make the sauce by heating all the ingredients in a small saucepan. Season with salt and black pepper and serve in slices, piping hot, with the sauce on the side.

Serves 4

4 red peppers

4 baby leeks, sliced

a few sprigs
fresh thyme

2 garlic cloves, sliced

a handful of fresh
basil leaves

1 teaspoon vegetable
bouillon stock powder

2 tablespoons
tomato Passata

6 sheets filo pastry
(30 x 20cm/12 x 8in)

1 egg, beaten

for the sauce

300ml (½ pint)
tomato Passata

1 teaspoon
ground cumin

1 teaspoon
ground coriander

1 tablespoon chopped
fresh coriander

1–2 teaspoons
vegetable bouillon
stock powder

salt and freshly ground
black pepper

per serving:
239 kcal/7.3g fat

Asparagus and Black Bean Pancakes

These delicious low-fat pancakes with a tasty filling are baked in the oven.

Serves 4

for the pancake batter

50g (2oz) plain flour

pinch of salt

1 egg

150ml (¼ pint) skimmed milk

1 tablespoon finely chopped fresh chervil

a little vegetable oil (to line the pan)

for the filling

225g (8oz) thin asparagus spears, trimmed and sliced diagonally

4 spring onions, finely sliced

2 tablespoons salted black beans, soaked overnight in cold water and drained

175g (6oz) fresh beansprouts

1 x 225g (8oz) tin water chestnuts, sliced

1 tablespoon Hoisin sauce

150ml (¼ pint) hot water

per serving:

125 kcal/2.4g fat

Step one Sift the flour and salt into a bowl. Make a well in the centre and add the egg and a little of the milk. Whisk to make a thick paste. Slowly add the remaining milk and the chervil, beating until smooth. Let stand for 20–30 minutes.

Step two Plunge the asparagus pieces into a pan of boiling salted water for 2 minutes, drain and plunge in cold water.

Step three Preheat a non-stick wok or frying pan until hot, add the spring onions and stir-fry for 1 minute. Add the beans, together with the asparagus, beansprouts and water chestnuts.

Step four Mix the Hoisin sauce with the water and pour over the vegetables and toss thoroughly, cooking for a further 2 minutes. Remove from the heat and allow to cool. Preheat the oven to 200°C/400°F/gas 6.

Step five Preheat a non-stick frying pan over medium heat with a little oil in it, then wipe out the pan with kitchen paper, taking care not to burn your fingers. Whisk the batter well, then add 2 tablespoons to the pan, tilting the pan to allow the batter to coat the base. Cook briskly for 30 seconds, then loosen the edges with a wooden spatula, flip the pancake over and cook the other side for 15 seconds, and slide onto a plate. Repeat until all the mixture is used, adding oil to the pan and wiping out after every 2 pancakes.

Step six When the pancakes are cool enough to handle, place 2 tablespoons of filling inside each one. Fold in both sides approximately 4cm (1½in), then roll into a spring-roll shape. Set in an ovenproof dish. Bake, uncovered, for 15–20 minutes.

Step seven Serve hot with noodles, rice or on a bed of stir-fried mixed vegetables.

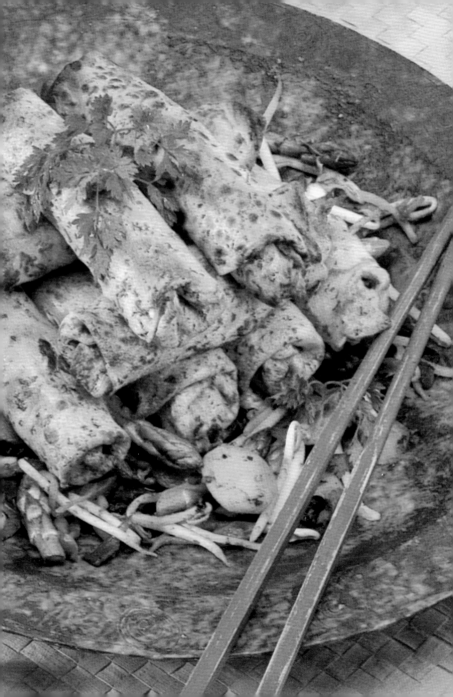

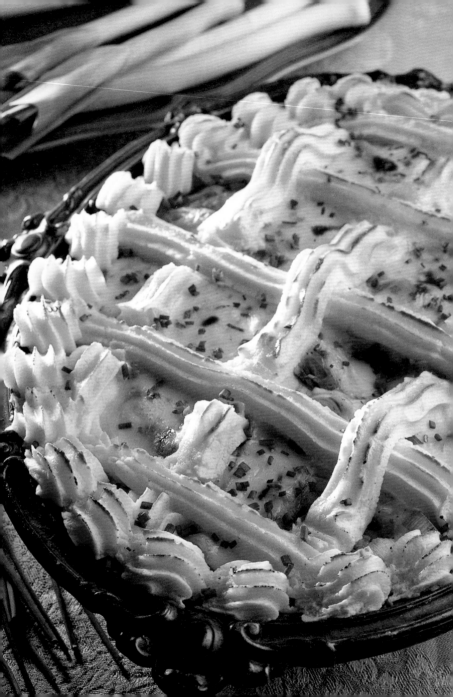

Onion, Potato and Fennel Bake

Potatoes and fennel make a great combination. Use a piping bag to spread the potato into the dish and create a lattice top for decoration.

Step one Preheat the oven to 200°C/400°F/gas 6.

Step two Boil the potatoes in salted water until cooked. Drain well and mash with a potato masher, adding the skimmed milk until the mixture is lump-free.

Step three Preheat a non-stick pan over medium heat. Add the fennel and dry-fry until it starts to colour. Remove the fennel from the pan and set aside. Add the onions, leeks and garlic to the pan and cook over high heat until they start to colour.

Step four Heat the milk and stock powder in a pan until boiling. Slake the cornflour with a little water and add to the milk, stirring continuously to prevent any lumps forming. Mix in the Cheddar and chives and season with salt and black pepper.

Step five Place the mashed potatoes in a piping bag. In an ovenproof dish, place alternate layers of piped potato, sauce and onion mixture, topping it off with a layer of potatoes piped in a lattice pattern.

Step six Bake for 20–25 minutes until browned and crisp on top. Garnish with a few snipped chives and serve with vegetables or salad.

Serves 4

675g (1½ lb) potatoes, peeled and chopped

2 tablespoons skimmed milk

1 large bulb fennel, thinly sliced

2 medium onions, finely sliced

4 leeks, washed and sliced

2 garlic cloves, crushed

600ml (1 pint) skimmed milk

2 teaspoons vegetable bouillon powder

2 tablespoons cornflour

50g (2oz) low-fat Cheddar

2 tablespoons snipped fresh chives, plus extra to garnish

salt and freshly ground black pepper

per serving:
299 kcal/3.1g fat

Tagliatelle with Sun-dried Tomato and Coriander Pesto

For the best pesto sauce ever, always use the freshest herbs you can find. Sun-dried tomatoes that are not packed in oil, used here, pack a punch of pure, unadulterated flavour without all the calories of the oil.

Serves 4

65g (2½oz) sun-dried tomatoes (non-oil variety)

2 garlic cloves, crushed

1 tablespoon ground coriander seeds

2 tablespoons chopped fresh coriander, plus a few extra leaves, to garnish

300ml (½ pint) tomato Passata

225g (8oz) tagliatelle

salt and freshly ground black pepper

per serving:
234 kcal/3.1g fat

Step one Place all the ingredients except the pasta in a food processor and blend until smooth. Season to taste with salt and black pepper.

Step two Cook the pasta in plenty of boiling salted water until tender, and drain.

Step three Heat the tomato pesto in a pan for 2–3 minutes. Add the cooked pasta and toss to coat thoroughly. Reheat, garnish with fresh coriander leaves and serve immediately.

For a video masterclass on making fresh pasta, go to www.mykitchentable.co.uk/videos/makingpasta

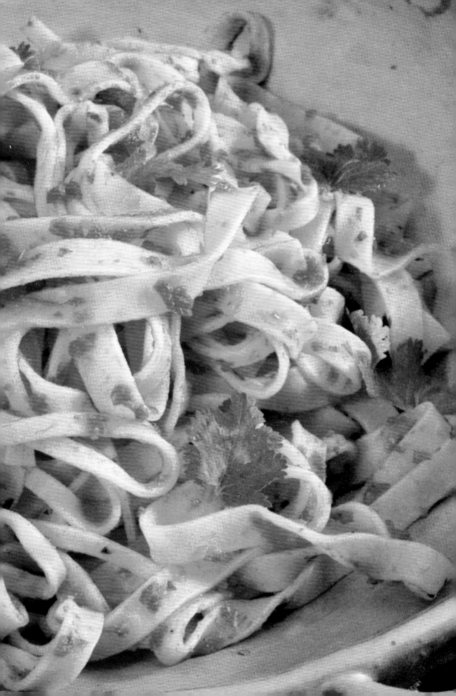

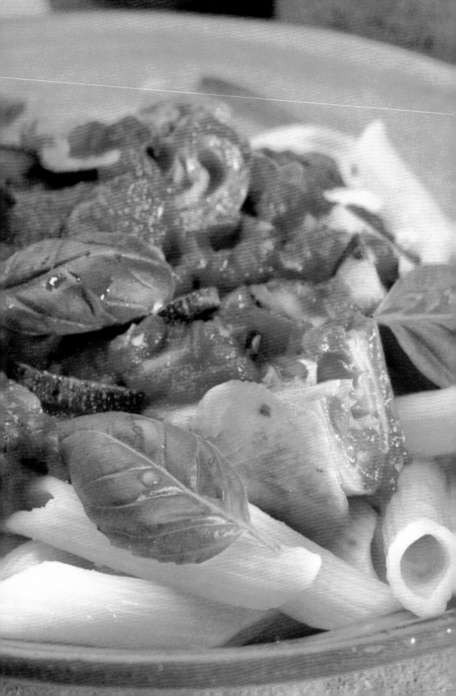

Penne with Artichokes, Chilli and Courgette

If you have a glut of courgettes in your garden, here is a healthy and delicious way to use some of them up.

Step one Cook the pasta in plenty of boiling salted water until tender, then drain.

Step two Meanwhile, make the sauce by dry-frying the onion and garlic in a non-stick pan over medium heat until soft. Add the courgette strips, artichoke hearts and chilli. Cook for a further 2–3 minutes, stirring regularly.

Step three Add the tomato Passata and the fresh basil. Season to taste with salt and black pepper and gently simmer until the sauce thickens.

Step four Place the pasta on a warmed serving dish and pour over the sauce. Garnish with a few whole basil leaves and serve with a crisp salad.

Serves 4

225g (8oz) penne pasta

for the sauce

1 red onion, finely diced

2 garlic cloves, crushed

2 young courgettes, cut into matchsticks

1 x 425g (15oz) tin artichoke hearts, drained and cut in half

1 small red chilli, finely sliced

300ml (½ pint) Passata

1 tablespoon chopped fresh basil, plus a few whole leaves, to garnish

salt and freshly ground black pepper

per serving:
276 kcal/3.9g fat

Chilli Pasta Bake

This rich tomato bake has a hint of chilli. If you prefer, you can omit the chilli and substitute a chopped red pepper.

Serves 4

225g (8oz) pasta shapes

2 courgettes, diced

2 medium leeks, washed and diced

2 garlic cloves, crushed

1 red chilli, seeded and finely chopped

1 tablespoon chopped fresh oregano

1 tablespoon chopped fresh parsley

600ml (1 pint) tomato Passata

2 tablespoons grated Parmesan

3 tablespoons low-fat natural yoghurt

salt and freshly ground black pepper

per serving:

250 kcal/3.3g fat

Step one Preheat the oven to 190°C/375°F/gas 5.

Step two Cook the pasta in boiling salted water until tender, then drain.

Step three In a large, non-stick pan, dry-fry the courgette, leeks and garlic over medium heat for 2–3 minutes. Add the chilli, herbs and Passata. Stir in the cooked pasta and season to taste.

Step four Transfer the mixture to an ovenproof dish and sprinkle with Parmesan. Bake for 30–35 minutes or until golden brown.

Step five Just before serving, drizzle with the yoghurt. Serve with a crisp salad or crusty bread.

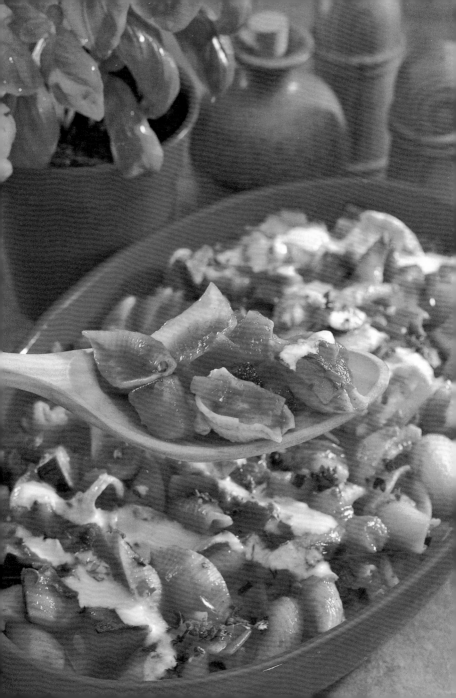

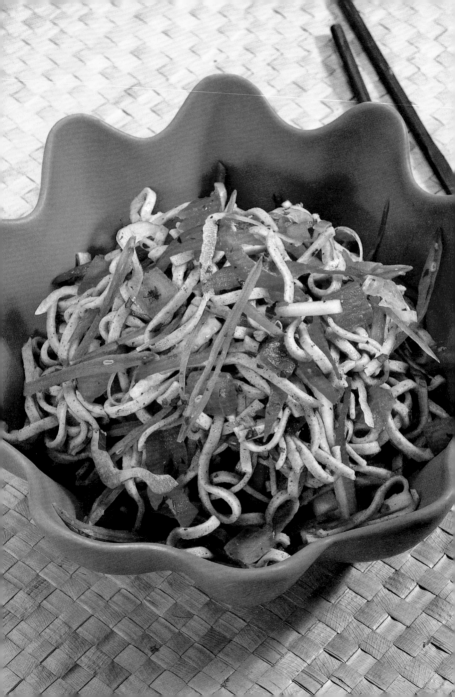

Hot Salad Noodles

Noodles have been part of the Chinese staple diet for more than 2,000 years – the ultimate Oriental fast food! Soba noodles are made using a blend of wheat flour and buckwheat flour and natural ingredients free from colourings and artificial flavourings. They have a distinctive, nutty flavour, rather like that of wholemeal pasta.

Step one Place the vegetables and chopped coriander in a large, non-metallic mixing bowl.

Step two Cook the noodles with the stock cube in plenty of boiling water, drain and add to the vegetables. Add the soy sauce and lemon juice and toss well.

Step three Reheat either in a microwave on full power for 2 minutes or in a steamer over boiling water for 2 minutes.

Step four Garnish with fresh coriander and serve hot.

Serves 4

1 small red onion, finely sliced

1 red pepper, seeded and finely sliced

1 fresh red chilli, seeded and finely chopped

½ cucumber, peeled and cut into matchsticks

4 ripe tomatoes, skinned, seeded and diced

115g (4oz) mangetout, cut into thin strips

2 tablespoons chopped fresh coriander

225g (8oz) soba noodles

1 vegetable stock cube

2 tablespoons light soy sauce

juice of 1 lemon

chopped fresh coriander, to garnish

per serving:
270 kcal/4.4g fat

167

Saffron Ravioli of Leek and Rocket with a Light Mustard Sauce

Making fresh pasta is simple, but keep the dough covered at all times.

Serves 6

for the pasta

good pinch of saffron

225g (8oz) double zero (00) pasta flour

½ teaspoon salt

1 egg, beaten

for the filling

4 baby leeks, chopped

1 teaspoon chopped fresh oregano

1 tablespoon chopped fresh flat-leaf parsley

50g (2oz) young rocket leaves, shredded

50g (2oz) quark (low-fat soft cheese)

salt

1 egg, beaten

for the sauce

600ml (1 pint) skimmed milk

1 onion, chopped

1 tablespoon vegetable stock powder

1 tablespoon cornflour

2 teaspoons coarse grain mustard

salt and freshly ground black pepper

per serving:

245 kcal/3.8g fat

Step one To make the pasta, add the saffron to 150ml (¼ pint) of water in a pan, bring to the boil and then allow to cool. Sift the flour and salt into a large mixing bowl. Make a well in the centre. Add the egg and some of the cooled saffron water and mix to a stiff dough, then turn out onto a floured board. Knead for 10 minutes. Wrap in clingfilm and chill for 1 hour.

Step two Meanwhile, make the filling by dry-frying the leeks until soft. Add the oregano and parsley. Remove from the heat and mix in the rocket and quark. Season well with salt.

Step three To make the ravioli, divide the dough in half. Roll out half on a floured surface or with a pasta machine until paper-thin. Place on a sheet of floured greaseproof paper. With a teaspoon, place blobs of filling over the dough at 2.5cm (1in) intervals. Brush between the fillings with beaten egg.

Step four Roll out the other half of the dough and use to cover the first, pressing down firmly between the fillings. Using a pastry wheel, cut out the individual ravioli, then dust each piece with flour, cover and set aside; allow 3–4 per person. Chill all the ravioli for 30 minutes.

Step five Now make the sauce by heating the milk, onion and stock powder in a non-stick pan. Slake the cornflour with a little cold water to form a paste and add slowly to the milk, stirring well until the milk comes to the boil. Cook for 2–3 minutes, add the mustard, season to taste and keep warm until using.

Step six Cook the ravioli in a large pan of boiling salted water for 2–3 minutes. Drain on kitchen paper. Arrange the ravioli on a serving plate and pour the hot sauce over it. Serve with vegetables or a mixed-leaf salad.

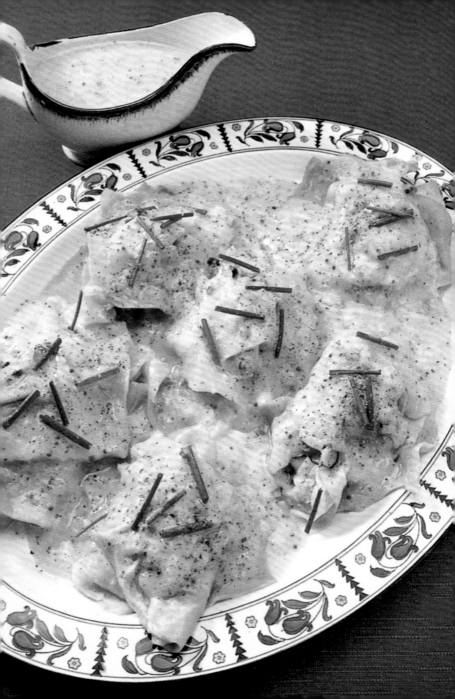

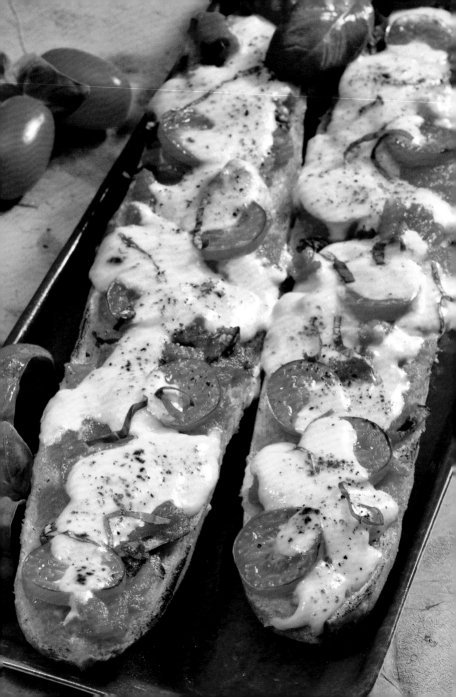

French-bread Margarita

An express, low-fat pizza for when you have little time to spare. However, do make sure you spread the mixture right up to the edges of the bread, or they may burn slightly when the baguette is returned to the grill.

Step one Preheat the grill to high.

Step two Lightly toast the bread on both sides. Then, using the cut side of the garlic, rub the top of the toasted bread, pressing the centre down.

Step three Empty the tinned tomatoes into a small bowl. Mix in the basil leaves and season well with salt and black pepper. Spread the mixture onto both pieces of bread, making sure it goes right up to the outside edges, and top with the sliced tomato.

Step four In a small bowl, mix together the salad dressing and cheese and spread on the top. Return to the grill until brown and bubbling.

Step five Garnish with the shredded basil leaves and serve immediately with a mixed salad.

Serves 1

1 small French baguette, split in half lengthways

1 garlic clove, peeled and cut in half

1 x 115g (4oz) tin chopped tomatoes

4–5 fresh basil leaves, plus a few extra, shredded, to garnish

8 cherry tomatoes, sliced

1 tablespoon low-fat salad dressing

1 tablespoon grated low-fat Cheddar

salt and freshly ground black pepper

per serving:
214 kcal/4g fat

Potatoes with Spinach

Tiny new potatoes are best for this dish, but you could also use larger ones or firm, old potatoes cut into 2.5cm (1in) dice.

Serves 4

2 teaspoons black mustard seeds

1½ teaspoons ground coriander

¼ teaspoon chilli powder

2 large onions, sliced

2 garlic cloves, crushed

450g (1lb) potatoes, peeled and cut into dice

350g (12oz) frozen leaf spinach

2 tomatoes, chopped

150ml (¼ pint) vegetable stock

chopped fresh coriander, to garnish

per serving:
159 kcal/1.6g fat

Step one Preheat a non-stick pan on low heat. Add the mustard seeds. Cook over low heat for a few seconds until the seeds begin to 'pop'. Remove from the heat and add the coriander and chilli powder and mix well.

Step two Return to the heat, then add the onions and garlic and cook together for 3–5 minutes. Add the potatoes to the pan and dry-fry for 2–3 minutes.

Step three Add the spinach, tomatoes and the stock. Cover and gently cook for 20–30 minutes until the potatoes are tender and only a little liquid remains in the pan. Check the pan occasionally to ensure the mixture doesn't burn on the bottom, and add a little more liquid if necessary.

Step four Transfer the mixture to a hot serving dish. Just before serving, sprinkle the chopped coriander over the top.

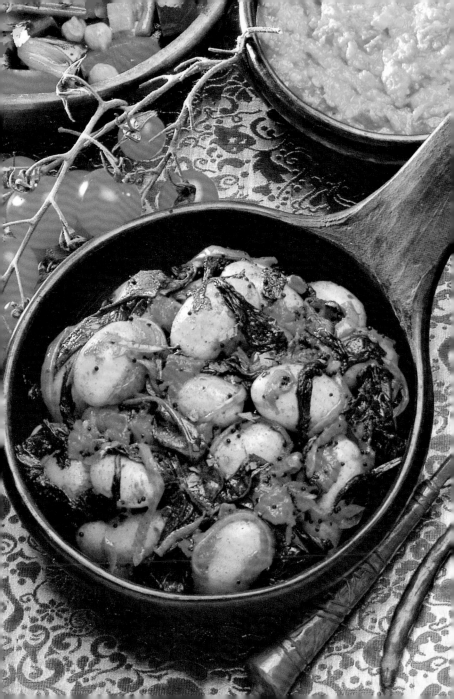

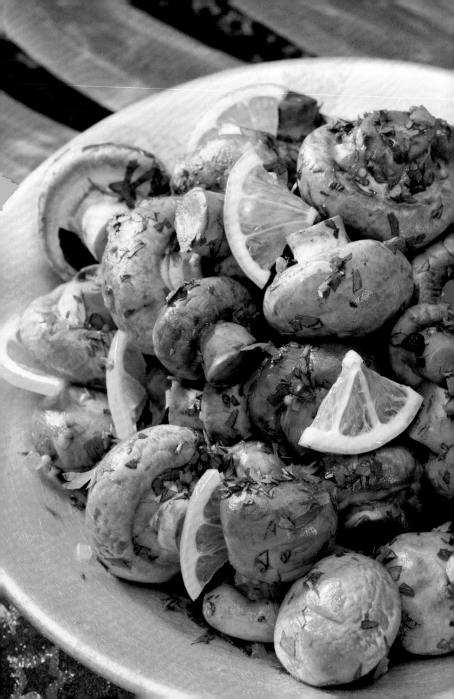

Mushrooms à la Grecque

Lemon and mushrooms make a wonderful combination and the perfect accompaniment to many fish dishes. Serve hot as a vegetable side dish or cold as a salad. You can even add a few fresh wild mushrooms for added flavour and colour.

Step one In a non-stick pan on medium heat, dry-fry the shallot until soft. Wipe the mushrooms with a damp cloth, add to the pan and cook for 1–2 minutes.

Step two Add the remaining ingredients, except the chopped parsley, and bring to the boil. Cover with a lid and remove the pan from the heat. Allow to cool.

Step three Before serving, remove the bay leaves and sprinkle with the parsley.

Serves 6

2 long shallots, finely chopped

1kg (2lb) small chestnut mushrooms

juice of 2 lemons

2 bay leaves

12 peppercorns

1 teaspoon coriander seeds

pinch of sea salt

2 tablespoons herb vinegar

1 tablespoon fresh apple juice

1 tablespoon chopped fresh parsley

per serving:
23 kcal/0.7g fat

Greek Salad

Instead of the traditional high-fat feta cheese and olives, I have used low-fat quark and black seedless grapes in this Greek-style salad. This makes it look similar to the real thing, and still taste delicious while keeping the calories and fat to a minimum.

Serves 4

1 crisp Romaine lettuce

1 cucumber, diced

6 ripe tomatoes, quartered

1 red onion, diced

1 green pepper, seeded and diced

225g (8oz) quark (low-fat soft cheese)

juice of 1 lemon

2 tablespoons chopped fresh parsley

salt and freshly ground black pepper

12 black seedless grapes, halved

for the dressing

150ml (¼ pint) apple juice

2 tablespoons white wine vinegar

1 tablespoon Dijon mustard

pinch of sugar

salt and freshly ground black pepper

Step one Combine all the salad vegetables in a large bowl.

Step two Using two dessertspoons, shape the quark into small balls. Place on a plate and season with salt and black pepper. Drizzle over the lemon juice and sprinkle with parsley.

Step three Arrange the salad on four individual plates. Place some quark on top of each salad, and scatter with the grapes.

Step four Combine all the dressing ingredients in a small bowl. Just before serving, pour the dressing over the salad.

Step five Serve with a jacket potato and natural yoghurt mixed with chives.

per serving:

101 kcal/1.1g fat

Have you made this recipe? Tell us what you think at
www.mykitchentable.co.uk/blog

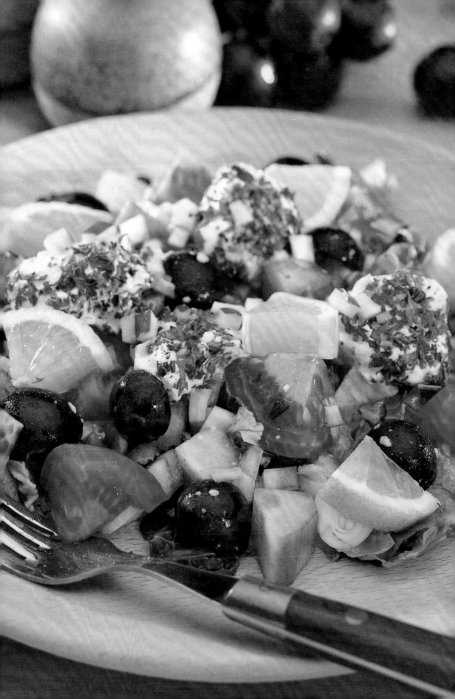

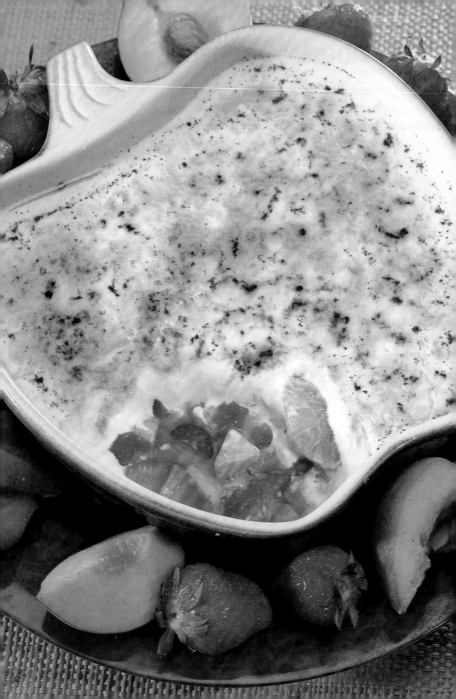

Fruit Brûlée

You can use any assortment of fruit for this sweet. Oranges, grapes and apples form a good base; pears, plums, raspberries, strawberries and redcurrants all provide a contrast in flavour and texture. Even in winter, a few frozen raspberries can be used, but frozen strawberries are not recommended as they are too moist.

Step one First, prepare your chosen fruit. Peel oranges, using a small, serrated knife, and cut out the segments. Wash grapes, cut them in half and remove the pips. Peel and dice apples and pears. Remove the stones from plums and cut into pieces. Wash fresh redcurrants, and wash and hull raspberries and strawberries. If using apples and pears, toss the dice in the lemon juice.

Step two Drain all the fruit well so that it is quite dry. Place the fruit in an ovenproof dish and chill.

Step three Preheat the grill until it is very hot.

Step four Just before you place the dish under the grill, spread the yoghurt over the fruit and sprinkle the sugar on top. (It is important that this is done immediately before grilling, otherwise the sugar melts and does not caramelise.) Place the dish as high under the grill as possible and watch it all the time to see that the top caramelises evenly. Turn the dish, if necessary, and ensure that the sugar doesn't burn.

Step five Allow to cool, then chill before serving.

Serves 4

450g (1lb) fresh fruit, such as oranges, grapes, apples, pears, plums, redcurrants, raspberries or strawberries

1–2 tablespoons lemon juice (for apples and pears only)

450g (16fl oz) 0 per cent fat or low-fat Greek-style yoghurt

4–5 tablespoons demerara or palm sugar

per serving:

176 kcal/0.3g fat

Fresh Mango and Lime Sorbet

Sorbet, while always low in fat, can be high in calories, as glucose syrup is often used to give it a smooth and creamy taste. Here, I have kept the calorie content to a minimum, resulting in a fresh, light dessert that resembles granita.

Serves 8

100g (4oz) caster sugar

2 large ripe mangoes

zest and juice of 2 limes

1 egg white

fresh lychees, to decorate

per serving:

80 kcal/0.2g fat

Step one In a pan, dissolve the sugar in 300ml (½ pint) water and bring to the boil. Remove from the heat and leave it to cool.

Step two Peel the mangoes and remove the flesh from the stone. Place in a food processor with the lime zest (reserve a little zest) and juice and blend to form a purée.

Step three Mix the purée with the cooled syrup and pour into a shallow freezer container. Cover and freeze for about 3 hours until mushy.

Step four Whisk the egg white until stiff. Fold into the loosened sorbet. Re-freeze for 4 hours until firm.

Step five Remove from the freezer and place in the refrigerator for 20 minutes to allow the sorbet to thaw slightly before serving. Slit open the lychees and use to decorate the sorbet along with the reserved zest.

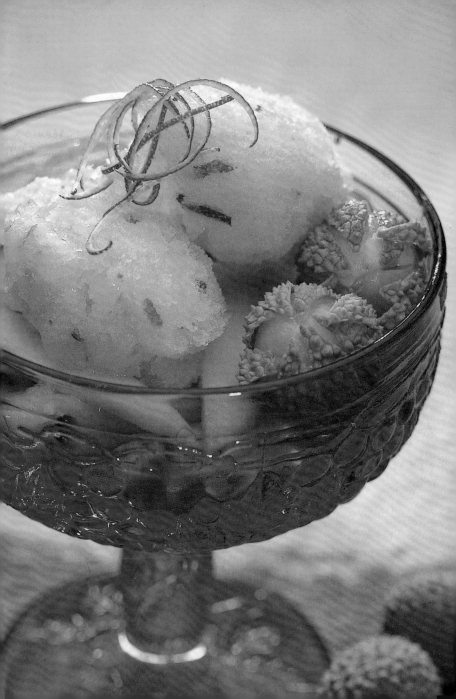

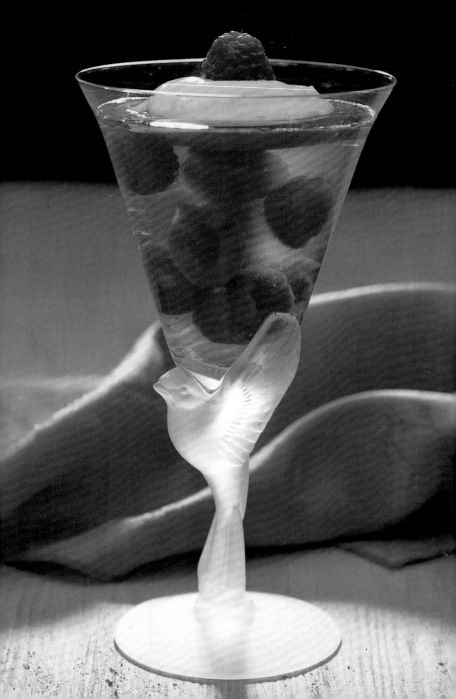

Sparkling Wine Jelly

This very pretty dessert offers another way to enjoy fresh fruit in season. Elegantly presented in a wine glass, no one will miss the calorie-heavy cream that so predictably accompanies fresh fruit.

Step one Sprinkle the gelatine over 3 tablespoons of water and allow to stand until spongy. Dissolve the gelatine over a pan of hot water or place in the microwave for 20–30 seconds and then stir until dissolved.

Step two Place the fruit squash, wine and 100ml (3½fl oz) water in a large jug and stir in the dissolved gelatine.

Step three Reserve a few raspberries for decoration and divide the remainder between four glasses. Fill the glasses with a little of the jelly. Place the glasses in the refrigerator for about 20 minutes until the jelly has set.

Step four When set, pour in the remaining jelly. (Doing this in two stages sets the raspberries at the bottom of the glass, but if time is short, you can top up the glasses immediately). Chill the jellies for about 2 hours until set.

Step five Top with a little yoghurt and the reserved raspberries.

In this recipe, when you add the gelatine to the jug containing the wine, the wine will fizz. For this reason, be sure to add the gelatine slowly and make sure that the jug is large enough to avoid any overspill.

Serves 4

1 x 11g (¼ oz) packet gelatine

3 tablespoons concentrated summer fruit squash

450ml (¾ pint) sparkling rosé wine

75g (3oz) raspberries

2 tablespoons 0 per cent fat or low-fat Greek-style yoghurt

per serving:
95 kcal/0.1g fat

Strawberry and Lime Pavlova

Here's proof that a low-calorie, low-fat dessert can still be high impact on flavour and presentation.

Serves 8

for the meringue

6 egg whites

350g (12oz) caster sugar

for the filling

225g (8oz) 0 per cent fat or low-fat Greek-style yoghurt

450g (1lb) fresh strawberries or other soft fruit, hulled and sliced

1 lime

per serving:

211 kcal/0.1g fat

Step one Preheat the oven to 140°C/275°F/gas 1. Line two baking sheets with non-stick baking parchment.

Step two Make the meringue by whisking the egg whites in a very clean, dry bowl with an electric whisk for 4–5 minutes until thick. Whisk in the caster sugar a tablespoon at a time, allowing 20 seconds in-between each one, until all the sugar is combined.

Step three Place the meringue in a large piping bag with a star nozzle. Pipe a disc, 30cm (12in) in diameter, onto the baking parchment of one baking sheet and pipe another disc, 20cm (8in) in diameter, onto the other. Place in the oven for approximately 2 hours or until the meringue has dried out and starts to colour. Remove from oven and allow to cool.

Step four Peel away the non-stick baking parchment and place the large meringue on a serving dish. Spread with yoghurt and cover with sliced strawberries. Place the smaller meringue on top and decorate with the remaining strawberries.

Step five Grate the zest of the lime with a fine grater and reserve. Slice the lime very thinly and tuck the slices in around the strawberries to decorate the meringue. Sprinkle the finely grated zest over the whole thing and serve.

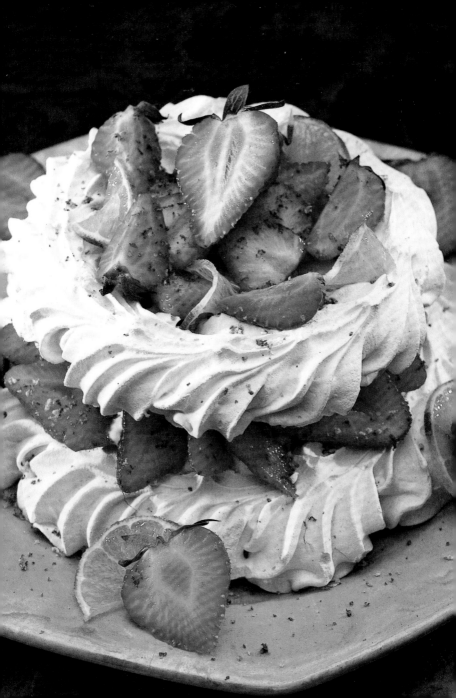

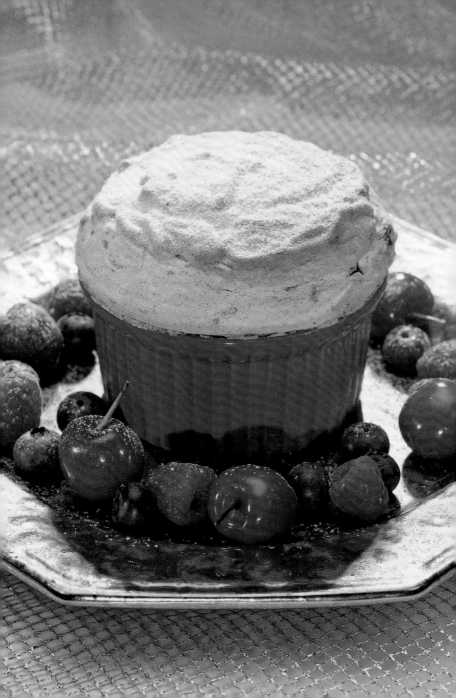

Quick Forest-fruit Soufflés

This simple but spectacular hot dessert has a very light texture and is a definite favourite of mine. If you have any extra fruit, you can combine it with a little sweet sherry and sugar to make a fruit compote to serve alongside the soufflés.

Step one Preheat the oven to 200°C/400°F/gas 6.

Step two Lightly grease four 50g (2oz) ramekins with a little margarine, then dust lightly with caster sugar and set aside.

Step three Place the fruit and the caster sugar in a small saucepan and gently simmer for 10–15 minutes until the fruit has reduced to a thick paste. Pour into a bowl and allow to cool.

Step four In a clean bowl, whisk the egg whites on full speed, adding only a pinch of caster sugar initially. Once the whites start to peak, gradually add the remaining sugar, using 1 dessertspoon at a time, allowing 10 seconds between each addition. Continue whisking until all the sugar is added.

Step five Place a dessertspoon of fruit into the base of each ramekin. Gently fold the egg whites into the remaining fruit purée. Pile into the ramekins, smoothing the tops and sides with a palette knife. The mixture should stand above the dishes.

Step six Place the ramekins in the oven and bake for 5–6 minutes. Once cooked, serve the soufflés immediately – they will start to collapse as soon as they come out of the oven.

Serves 4

a little margarine, for greasing

225g (8oz) frozen forest fruits, such as blackberries and raspberries

25g (1oz) caster sugar

for the meringue

3 egg whites

150g (5oz) caster sugar

fresh fruit, to decorate

per serving:

187 kcal/0.1g fat

Pineapple and Papaya Salad with Lime and Ginger Yoghurt

This makes a refreshing finish to a hot and spicy meal. You can substitute any fresh fruits, but try to aim for a mixture of flavours and textures. The fruits can be prepared in advance, but the yoghurt should be mixed just before serving as it may separate if allowed to stand.

Serves 4

1 large ripe pineapple

2 ripe papaya

2 tablespoons sesame seeds (optional)

for the yoghurt

1 vanilla pod

300ml (½ pint) 0 per cent fat or low-fat Greek-style yoghurt

zest and juice of 1 lime

1 x 2.5cm (1in) piece fresh ginger, finely chopped

caster sugar, to taste

per serving:

115 kcal/4g fat

Step one Prepare the pineapple by slicing off the top and bottom with a sharp knife. Stand the fruit upright and cut away the skin from top to bottom, slicing around it to leave a barrel-like shape. Cut the pineapple in half and then into slices.

Step two Using a sharp knife, cut away the skin from the papaya, then slice each papaya in half lengthways. Remove the black seeds from the centres and discard. Cut the fruits into long slices and arrange with the pineapple slices in alternate layers on a serving plate.

Step three Place the sesame seeds (if using) in a non-stick frying pan and lightly toast over a low heat until browned, then scatter them over the pineapple and papaya slices.

Step four Split the vanilla pod down the centre with a sharp knife (see tip). Scrape out the seeds from the inside with the tip of the knife and place in a bowl. Add the yoghurt, lime juice, fresh ginger and sugar to taste. Mix well and serve together with the fruit salad.

Once you have removed the seeds from the vanilla pod, you can store the pod in a sealed jar of caster sugar. After a couple of weeks the sugar will take on the flavour and fragrance of the vanilla.

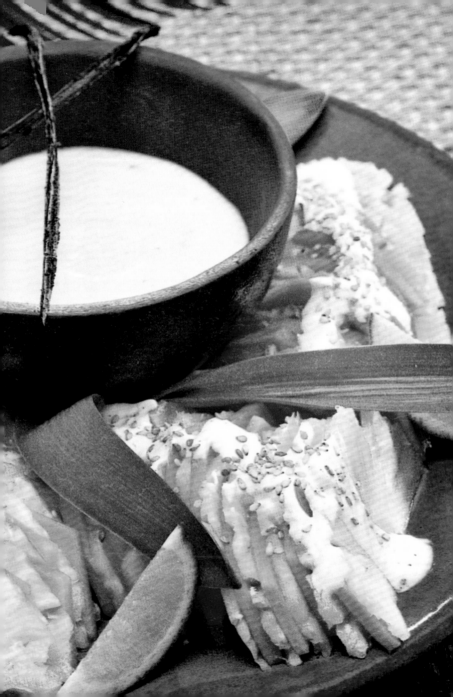

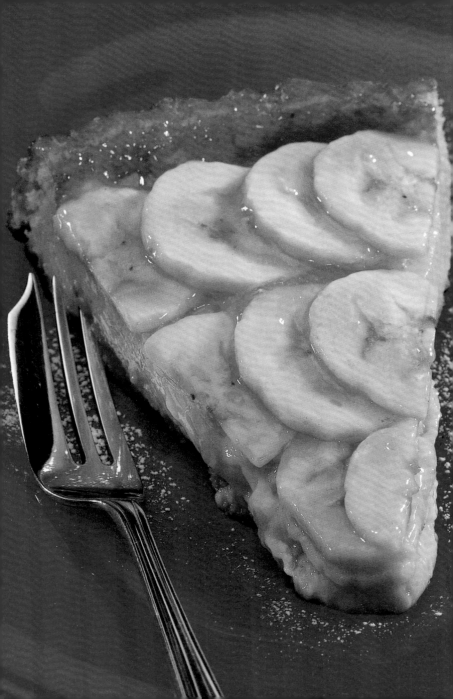

Banana and Custard Tart

Here, the sponge base can be frozen in advance. The frozen base can then be filled with the hot custard, which cools the custard more quickly.

Step one Preheat the oven to 180°C/350°F/gas 4. Lightly grease a 20cm (8in) non-stick flan case with a little oil, then dust with caster sugar, discarding the excess.

Step two To make the sponge base, whisk together the eggs and sugar for several minutes until pale and thick in consistency. Sift the flour and then, using a metal spoon, carefully fold the sifted flour into the egg mixture, followed by the vanilla essence.

Step three Pour into the flan case, level off with a knife and bake in the centre of the oven for 20 minutes until golden brown. Loosen the sponge from the flan case with a palette knife, then allow to cool.

Step four Using a sharp, serrated knife, cut away a 1cm (½in) layer of sponge from the centre of the flan case to make a deeper 'well'. Then use a spoon to scrape away any crumbs to leave a smooth surface.

Step five To make the filling, mix the custard powder and sugar with a little of the milk to form a paste. Pour the remaining milk into a pan. Split the vanilla pod lengthways with a sharp knife, scrape away the seeds and add to the milk in the saucepan. Heat until boiling, pour onto the custard powder and mix well. Pour the mixture back into the pan and bring to the boil until the mixture thickens. Pour into the flan case and allow to cool.

Step six Peel and slice the bananas into a bowl. Pour the lemon juice over the bananas and gently toss. Then arrange the bananas on top of the flan. Heat the apricot jam and brush over the bananas to form a glaze. Serve immediately.

Serves 8

for the sponge base

2 eggs

75g (3oz) caster sugar

75g (3oz) self-raising flour

1 teaspoon vanilla essence

for the filling

1 tablespoon low-fat custard powder

1 tablespoon caster sugar

250ml (8fl oz) skimmed milk

1 vanilla pod

2 large bananas

juice of ½ lemon

2 tablespoons sieved apricot jam

per serving:

184 kcal/1.8g fat

Lime Cheesecake Ice Cream

Light evaporated milk forms the base of this luxurious, creamy dessert. It is very important that the milk is completely chilled overnight in order to achieve the thick foam once whisked.

Serves 6

4 large limes

2 x 175g (6oz) tins light evaporated milk, chilled overnight

1 vanilla pod

75g (3oz) caster sugar

225g (8oz) virtually fat-free fromage frais

115g (4oz) quark (low-fat cheese)

3 x 90 per cent fat-free ginger biscuits, crushed, to decorate

per serving:

150 kcal/1.3g fat

Step one Finely grate the lime zest from all 4 limes into a mixing bowl and add the evaporated milk. Using an electric mixer, whisk the evaporated milk on high speed until thick and doubled in volume.

Step two Cut the limes in half and squeeze out the juice into a small pan. Split the vanilla pod lengthways, using a sharp knife, and scrape out the black seeds from the centre and add to the pan, along with the sugar. Gently heat, stirring until the sugar has dissolved.

Step three Whisk the hot syrup into the milk until fully combined. Carefully fold in the fromage frais and quark and pour into a plastic freezer container. Cover and freeze for 4–5 hours until firm.

Step four Remove from the freezer 10 minutes before serving. Serve 2–3 scoops per serving, sprinkled with the crushed ginger biscuits.

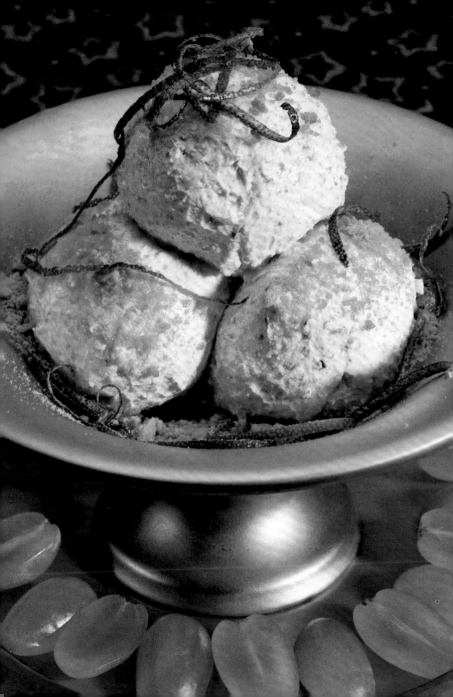

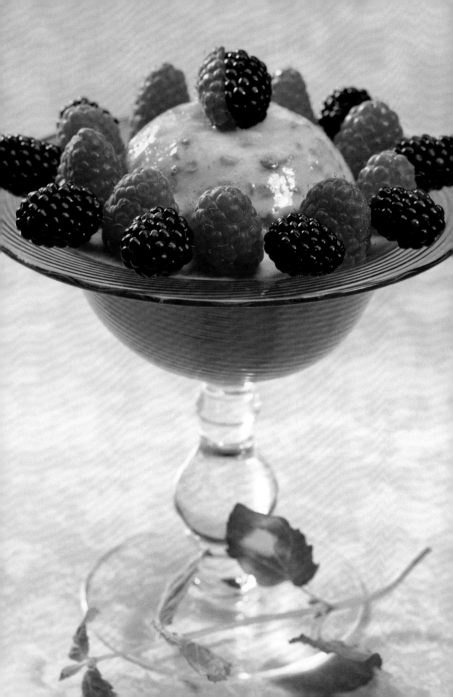

Raspberry Bavarois

There are many different types of fromage frais and low-fat yoghurts available that can be used for this type of recipe. However, good-quality varieties tend to have a richer texture and not such sharp flavours. Make this recipe in advance and chill until ready to serve.

Step one Soak the gelatine in cold water in a bowl for 2–3 minutes until it becomes soft. Place the bowl and heat it either over a pan of boiling water or in a microwave on High for 1 minute until liquid.

Step two Add the fromage frais and Grenadine to the gelatine and mix together thoroughly. Carefully fold in the raspberries with a little sugar to taste and blend again until combined.

Step three Whisk the egg whites until stiff and fold into the mixture.

Step four Spoon into individual glasses or place in a glass bowl and decorate with extra raspberries, blackberries and mint leaves.

Serves 4

6 sheets leaf gelatine

450g (1lb) virtually fat-free fromage frais

2 tablespoons Grenadine

275g (10oz) fresh raspberries

caster sugar, to taste

3 egg whites

to decorate

a few raspberries and blackberries

mint leaves

per serving:

107 kcal/0.4g fat

Banana Split with Hot Chocolate Sauce

A dessert to die for! Although low in fat, this dessert makes up for it in calories, so make sure you adapt your main meals accordingly.

Serves 4

for the hot sauce

1 tablespoon high-quality cocoa powder

300ml (½ pint) semi-skimmed milk

2 teaspoons cornflour

1 tablespoon caster sugar

for the banana split

4 small ripe bananas

2 tablespoons lemon juice

225g (8oz) fresh raspberries

8 scoops low-fat ice cream or other similar iced dessert

per serving:

199 kcal/4.4g fat

Step one In a small pan, heat the cocoa powder with the milk, whisking continuously.

Step two Slake the cornflour with a little cold milk and whisk into the hot milk. Simmer for 1 minute as the sauce thickens, then add sugar to taste. Keep warm over a low heat.

Step three Peel the bananas, slice in half lengthways and place in a serving dish. Sprinkle with the lemon juice to prevent them turning brown.

Step four Divide the raspberries between the four dishes. Place 2 scoops of low-fat ice cream or iced dessert on top of the raspberries and then pour the chocolate sauce over. Serve immediately.

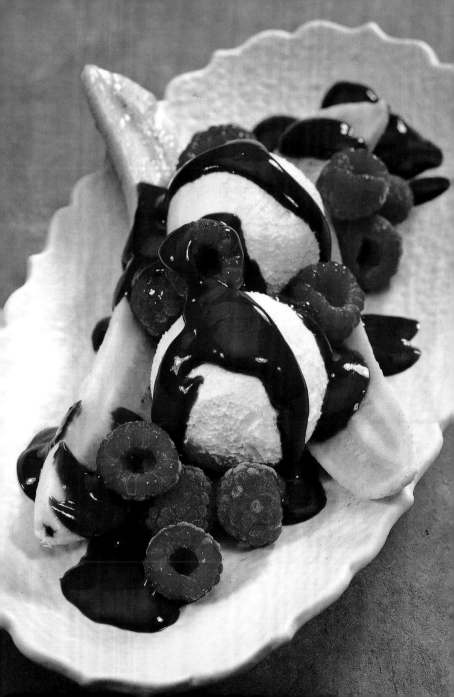

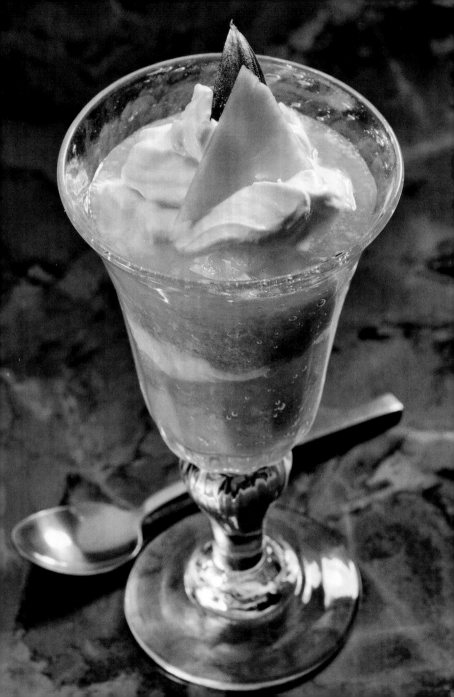

Apricot and Almond Syllabub

Syllabub dates back to as early as the sixteenth century. Traditionally, it was made by sweetening rich milk or cream with sugar and then lightly curdling it with wine. Thanks to low-fat yoghurt, this modern version offers only a fraction of the calories, but all the pleasure of the original.

Step one Place the apricots and lime zest and juice into a small pan and cover with water. Bring to the boil and simmer until soft and virtually all the water has evaporated. Using a fork, mash the apricots until smooth.

Step two Beat the yoghurt into the apricot mixture, add the liqueur and sweeten to taste with a little sugar.

Step three Whisk the egg white to stiff peaks and gently fold into the mixture. Spoon into a glass, layering it with a little extra yoghurt if liked. Chill until required. Decorate with a wedge of lime to serve.

Serves 1

25g (1oz) dried apricots

zest and juice of 1 lime

4–5 tablespoons 0 per cent fat or low-fat Greek-style yoghurt, plus a little extra to serve (optional)

2 teaspoons Amaretto liqueur

caster sugar, to taste

1 egg white

wedge of lime, to decorate

per serving:

174 kcal/1.4g fat

For more recipes from My Kitchen Table, sign up for our newsletter at
www.mykitchentable.co.uk/newsletter

Caramel Coffee Pears with Vanilla Sauce

Choose firm pears, without any bruising, as the discoloration caused by bruising will show once the pear has been peeled. The vanilla sauce can be made in advance and stored with a disc of non-stick baking parchment on the top to avoid a skin forming.

Serves 4

4 large firm pears

2 tablespoons lemon juice

115g (4oz) caster sugar

50ml (2fl oz) coffee

for the sauce

300ml (½ pint) semi-skimmed milk

1 vanilla pod

2 teaspoons cornflour

sugar, to taste, plus extra for dusting

per serving:

255 kcal/1.4g fat

Step one Peel the pears and cut in half lengthways. Scoop out the cores with a spoon and rub the surface of the pears with the lemon juice. Place the pears in a large bowl and sprinkle the sugar over to coat.

Step two Preheat a non-stick pan over low heat. Add the pears, placing them face down in the pan. Cook gently until the sugar starts to caramelise, then add the coffee and continue cooking until the pears soften.

Step three In the meantime, make the sauce by heating the milk in a saucepan. Split the vanilla pod lengthways, scrape out the seeds and add them to the milk along with the pod. Slake the cornflour with a little cold water and whisk into the hot milk. Gently simmer to allow the sauce to thicken, and add a little sugar to taste.

Step four Arrange the pears in a serving dish and pour the sauce around them. Dust lightly with a little sugar and serve.

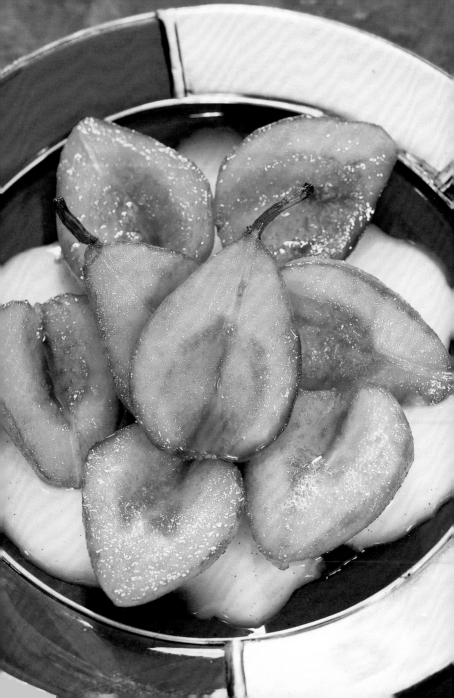

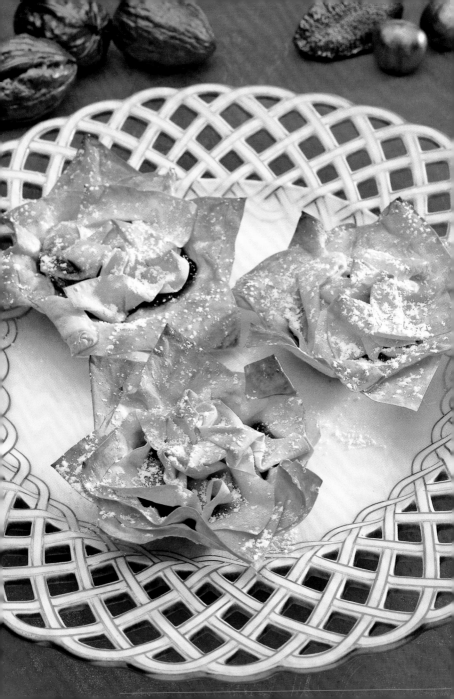

Filo Pastry Mince Pies

Here's an updated, lighter version of a traditionally calorie-laden Christmas treat.

Step one Preheat the oven to 190°C/375°F/gas 5.

Step two Stack the filo pastry sheets on top of one another on the worktop. Using scissors, cut the stack into 6 square-shaped sections, so that you end up with 36 individual squares.

Step three Take 6 non-stick patty tins. In each patty tin, place 4 individual filo pastry squares at slight angles to each other, brushing with beaten egg white in-between each layer. Then place half a tablespoonful of mincemeat in the centre of each pastry case.

Step four Brush the remaining 12 pastry squares with egg white and scrunch them up to make crinkly toppings for the pies. Place two scrunched-up squares on top of each portion of mincemeat.

Step five Bake for 10 minutes until the pastry is crisp and golden. Just before serving, dust the mince pies with a little icing sugar, if using.

Makes 6

6 sheets filo pastry (30cm x 20cm/ 12in x 8in)

1 egg white, beaten

3 tablespoons spicy fat-free mincemeat

icing sugar, to dust (optional)

per mince pie:

144 kcal/1.5g fat

Low-fat Christmas Pudding

This is an old faithful recipe that tastes even better than the full-fat original.

Serves 10

75g (3oz) each currants and sultanas

115g (4oz) raisins

4 tablespoons brandy, rum or beer

75g (3oz) glacé cherries, halved

75g (3oz) flour

1 teaspoon mixed spice

½ teaspoon ground cinnamon

50g (2oz) fresh breadcrumbs

50g (2oz) Muscovado or caster sugar

2 teaspoons gravy browning

grated zest of ½ lemon

grated zest of ½ orange

115g (4oz) grated apple

115g (4oz) finely grated carrot

1 tablespoon lemon juice

2 eggs

4 tablespoons skimmed milk

2 tablespoons molasses or cane-sugar syrup

4 tablespoons rum

per serving:
280 kcal/2.5g fat

Step one Soak the dried fruit in the brandy, rum or beer and leave overnight.

Step two When ready to make the pudding, slake the cherries gently in the flour and then add the mixed spice, cinnamon, breadcrumbs, sugar and gravy browning.

Step three Mix in the grated zest, apple and carrot, together with the lemon juice and the soaked fruit.

Step four Beat the eggs with the milk and molasses and gradually add to the mixture, stirring well. Mix together gently but thoroughly.

Step five Place in an ovenproof basin with a capacity of 1.2 litres (2 pints). To microwave the pudding, place an upturned plate over the basin and cook on High for 5 minutes. Leave to stand for 5 minutes, then cook for a further 5 minutes. If steaming the pudding, cover with foil or a pudding cloth, and then steam gently for 3 hours (this makes a moister pudding).

Step six After cooking, allow the pudding to cool and then wrap in foil. Leave in a cool, dry place until required.

Step seven Before reheating, pierce the pudding several times with a fork and pour some more rum over the top. Steam for 1–2 hours or microwave on High for 10 minutes.

You can deep-freeze this Christmas pudding, but do take care to thaw it thoroughly before reheating. If you prefer, you can use brandy instead of rum when you reheat it before serving.

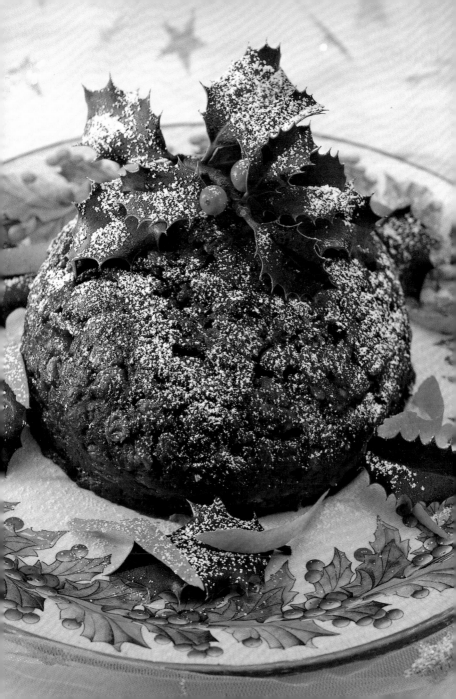

Apricot and Almond Syllabub 198–9
Arrabbiata prawns 134–5
asparagus
    and Black Bean Pancakes 156–7
    Soup, Cream of 6–7
Aubergine, Stuffed 146–7
Baked Salmon with Sweet Ginger 122–3
Baked Sea Bass with Dill and Lemon Sauce 120–1
banana
    and Custard Tart 190–1
    Split with Hot Chocolate Sauce 196–7
beef
    Boeuf à la Bourguignonne 84–5
    Cottage Pie with Leek and Potato Topping 80–1
    Minced Beef and Potato Pie 82–3
    Rich Spaghetti Bolognese 88–9
    Roast Beef with Yorkshire Pudding, Dry-roast Potatoes and Parsnips 92–3
    Tomato-braised with Oyster Mushrooms 90–1
    Wellingtons with Red Wine Sauce 86–7
    Blinis with Smoked Salmon and Horseradish Cream 40–1
Brûlée, Fruit 178–9
Caramel Coffee Pears with Vanilla Sauce 200–1
casserole
    Chicken with Peppers 54–5
    Chicken Winter 58–9
    Cauliflower and Basil Soup 20–1
    Celeriac and Nutmeg Soup 12–3
chicken 44–67
    and Pork Pâté with Spiced Plums 34–5
    Casserole with Peppers 54–5
    Caesar Salad 44–5

Coconut and Coriander 60–1
Jamaican Jerk 46–7
Lemon Roast with Fresh Herb Stuffing 66–7
Oven-baked Tikka Masala 64–5
Spicy Lemon 50–1
Stuffed Breast 52–3
Thai Breasts 48–9
Thai Curry 56–7
Tunisian 62–3
Winter Casserole 58–9
chilli
    Pasta Bake 164–5
    Prawn Couscous 138–9
chowder:
    Crab and Tomato 26–7
    Smoked Fish and Corn 28–9
Christmas Pudding 204–5
Coconut and Coriander Chicken 60–1
Cottage Pie with Leek and Potato Topping 80–1
Couscous, Chilli Prawn 138–9
crab
    and Tomato Chowder 26–7
    Bisque 24–5
Cream of Asparagus Soup 6–7
Cream of Wild Mushroom Soup 18–9
Curry, Thai Chicken 56–7
Dhansak, Leek and Courgette 150–1
Duck, Low-fat with Black Cherries 78–9
Filo Pastry Mince Pies 202–3
French Bread Margarita 170–1
Fruit Brûlée 178–9
Gammon with Pineapple Rice 96–7
ginger
    and Turkey Stir-fry 70–1
    and Watercress Soup 16–7
    Baked Salmon with Sweet Ginger 122–3
    Pineapple and Papaya Salad with Lime and Ginger Yoghurt 188–9
Greek Salad 176–7

Grilled Polenta with Wild Mushrooms 148–9
Guinea Fowl, Lemon-baked 76–7
Haddock Boats, Smoked 118–9
ham
    Pheasant Wrapped in Parma Ham with Red Wine 74–5
    Smoked Ham and Mushroom Coddle 102–3
Honey-roast Pork with Prune and Apple Stuffing 94–5
Hot Salad Noodles 166–7
Hummus, Sun-dried Tomato with Vegetables 38–9
Ice cream, Lime Cheesecake 192–3
Jamaican Jerk Chicken 46–7
Jelly, Sparkling Wine 182–3
lamb
    and Pepper Crumble 106–7
    Liver with Orange Sauce 112–3
    Moussaka 110–1
    Pot Roast 104–5
    Samosas with Dipping Sauce 114–5
    Steaks Boulangères 108–9
Lasagne, Salmon and Broccoli 128–9
leek
    and Courgette Dhansak 150–1
    Cottage Pie with Leek and Potato Topping 80–1
    Roasted Pepper and Leek Strudel 154–5
    Saffron Ravioli of Leek and Rocket 168–9
lemon
    and Caper-stuffed Peppers 30–1
    Pork with Capers 98–9
    Roast Chicken with Fresh Herb Stuffing 66–7
lime
    Cheesecake Ice Cream 192–3

Fresh Mango and Lime Sorbet 180–1

Pineapple and Papaya Salad 188–9

Tuna Roll-ups 130–1

Mackerel Salad Niçoise, Smoked 116–7

Mango and Lime Sorbet, Fresh 180–1

Minced Beef and Potato Pie 82–3

mushroom
à la Grecque 174–5
Cream of Wild Mushroom Soup 18–9
Grilled Polenta with Wild Mushrooms 148–9
Pheasant Breast with Wild Mushrooms 72–3
Smoked Ham and Mushroom Coddle 102–3
tomato-braised Beef with Oyster Mushrooms 90–1

noodles
Hot Salad 166–7
Pan-fried Tuna with Pepper Noodles 126–7
Thai Noodle Soup 14–5

Onion, Potato and Fennel Bake 158–9

Oven-baked Chicken Tikka Masala 64–5

Paella 136–7

Pancakes, Asparagus and Black Bean 156–7

Pan-fried Tuna with Pepper Noodles 126–7

pasta
Chilli Pasta Bake 164–5
Penne with Artichokes, Chilli and Courgette 162–3
Rich Spaghetti Bolognese 88–9
Tagliatelle with Sun-dried Tomato and Pesto 160–1

Pâté, Pork and Chicken with Spiced Plums 34–5

Pavlova, Strawberry and Lime 184–5

pears
Caramel Coffee Pears with Vanilla Sauce 200–1
Lemon- and Caper-stuffed 30–1

Penne with Artichokes, Chilli and Courgette 162–3

peppers
Chicken Casserole with 54–5
Double Soup of Red and Yellow 22–3
Lamb Pot Roast with Celery and 104–5
Roasted Pepper and Leek Strudel 154–5
Sweet Potato and Red Pepper Terrine 36–7
Sweetcorn and Red Pepper Soup 8–9

pheasant
Breast of with Wild Mushrooms 72–3
Wrapped in Parma Ham with Red Wine 74–5

pies
Cottage Pie with Leek and Potato Topping 80–1
Minced Beef and Potato 82–3
Seafood 132–3
The Easiest Vegetable Pie Ever 152–3

Pineapple and Papaya Salad 188–9

Polenta Grilled with Wild Mushrooms 148–9

pork
and Chicken Pâté with Spiced Plums 34–5
Honey-roast with Prune and Apple Stuffing 94–5
Lemon with Capers 98–9
Sage and Onion Roast 100–1

potatoes
Minced Beef and Potato Pie 82–3
Onion, Potato and Fennel Bake 158–9
Roast Beef with Yorkshire Pudding, Dry-roast Potatoes

and Parsnips 92–3
Sweet Potato and Red Pepper Terrine 36–7
with Spinach 172–3

prawn
Arrabbiata 134–5
Cocktail 42–3
Steamed Sesame Prawn Balls with Lime Dip 140–1

Quick Forest Fruit Soufflés 186–7

Raspberry Bavarois 194–5

Ravioli, Saffron Ravioli of Leek and Rocket with a Light Mustard Sauce 168–9

Rich Spaghetti Bolognese 88–9

Roast Beef with Yorkshire Pudding, Dry-roast Potatoes and Parsnips 92–3

Roasted Pepper and Leek Strudel 154–5

Saffron Ravioli of Leek and Rocket 168–9

Sage and Onion Roast Pork 100–1

salad
Chicken Caesar 44–5
Greek 176–7
Pineapple and Papaya with Lime and Ginger Yoghurt 188–9
Smoked Mackerel Niçoise 116–7

salmon
and Broccoli Lasagne 128–9
Blinis with Smoked Salmon and Horseradish Cream 40–1
with Sweet Ginger, Baked 122–3

Scallops with Carrot and Pink Ginger Pickle, Seared 142–3

Sea Bass with Dill and Lemon Sauce, Baked 120–1

Seafood Pie 132–3

smoked
Fish and Corn Chowder 28–9
Haddock Boats 118–9
Ham and Mushroom Coddle

102–3
Mackerel Salad Niçoise
116–7
Sorbet, Fresh Mango and Lime 180–1
Soufflés, Quick Forest Fruit 186–7
soups
Cauliflower and Basil 20–1
Celeriac and Nutmeg 12–3
Crab and Tomato Chowder 26–7
Crab Bisque 24–5
Cream of Asparagus 6–7
Cream of Wild Mushroom 18–9
Double Soup of Red and Yellow Peppers 22–3
Smoked Fish and Corn Chowder 28–9
Spring Vegetable 10–1
Sweetcorn and Red Pepper 8–9
Thai Noodle 14–5
Watercress and Ginger 16–7

Spaghetti Bolognese 88–9
Sparkling Wine Jelly 182–3
Spicy Lemon Chicken 50–1
Squid, Marinated Griddled 144–5
Steamed Sesame Prawn Balls with Lime Dip 140–1
Stir-fry, Turkey and Ginger 70–1
Strawberry and Lime Pavlova 184–5
Strudel, Roasted Pepper and Leek 154–5
Stuffed Aubergine 146–7
Stuffed Chicken Breast 52–3
Sun-dried Tomato Hummus with Roasted Summer Vegetables 38–9
Sweet Potato and Red Pepper Terrine 36–7
Syllabub, Apricot and Almond 198–9
Tagliatelle with Sun-dried Tomato 160–1
Tart, Banana and Custard

190–1
Terrine, Sweet Potato and Red Pepper 36–7
Thai
Chicken Breasts 48–9
Chicken Curry 56–7
Noodle Soup 14–5
tomato
-braised Beef with Oyster Mushrooms 90–1
Crab and Tomato Chowder 26–7
Hummus with Roasted Vegetables 38–9
Tagliatelle with Pesto 160–1
Trout and Spinach Paupiettes 124–5
tuna
Lime Tuna Roll-ups 130–1
Pan-fried Tuna with Pepper Noodles 126–7
Tunisian Chicken 62–3
turkey
and Pepper Stroganoff 68–9
and Ginger Stir-fry 70–1

10 9 8 7 6 5 4 3

Published in 2011 by Ebury Press, an imprint of Ebury Publishing
A Random House Group company

Recipes © Rosemary Conley Enterprises 2011
Photography © Peter Barry
Photography on p4 by Alan Olley © Ebury Press 2011
Book design © Ebury Press 2011

All recipes contained in this book first appeared in Rosemary Conley's *Low Fat Cookbook* (1999), *Low Fat Cookbook Two* (2000), *Eat Yourself Slim* (2002) and *Step by Step Low Fat Cookbook* (2007).

Rosemary Conley has asserted her right to be identified as the author of this Work in accordance with the Copyright, Designs and Patents Act 1988

The Random House Group Limited
Reg. No. 954009

Addresses for companies within the Random House Group can be found at www.randomhouse.co.uk

A CIP catalogue record for this book is available from the British Library

The Random House Group Limited supports the Forest Stewardship Council® (FSC®), the leading international forest certification organisation. All our titles that are printed on Greenpeace approved FSC® certified paper carry the FSC® logo. Our paper procurement policy can be found at www.randomhouse.co.uk/environment

To buy books by your favourite authors and register for offers visit www.randomhouse.co.uk

Printed and bound in the UK by Butler, Tanner and Dennis Ltd
Colour origination by AltaImage

Commissioning Editor: Muna Reyal
Assistant Editor: Joe Cottington
Project Editor: Constance Novis
Designer: Lucy Stephens
Food Stylists: Dean Simpole-Clarke and Chris Sismore
Copy Editor: Emily Hatchwell
Production: Rebecca Jones

ISBN: 9780091944803

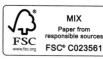